Plain & Simple Guide
to Therapeutic
Massage & Bodywork
Certification

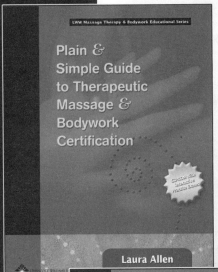
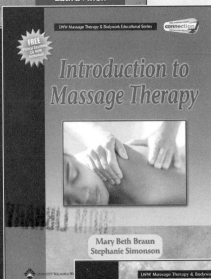
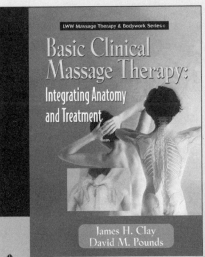
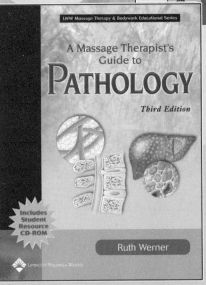
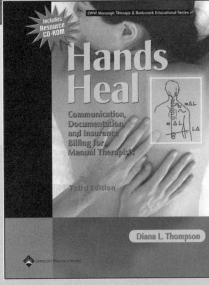
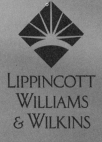

Resource CD-ROM

for

Plain & Simple Guide to Therapeutic Massage & Bodywork Certification

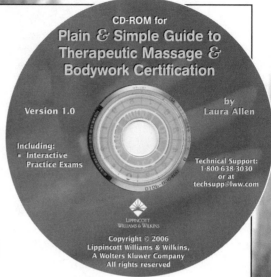

As a bonus for you, Lippincott Williams & Wilkins has included an interactive CD-ROM to enhance your learning and comprehension!

This resource is the perfect tool to help you prepare for the National Certification Examination, state or local exams, or tests in school. Practice taking the exam on a computer just like the National Certification Examination.

The CD-ROM includes:

- Three complete practice tests with 170 questions each mimic the National Certification Examination.

- Two options for taking the practice tests: study mode and test mode. Study mode allows you to immediately see if you answered correctly while test mode provides a score and the opportunity to review the correct answers at the end of the test.

- Rationales for the correct answer so you can understand the reasoning behind the correct answer.

For technical support, contact 1-800-638-3030 or techsupp@lww.com.

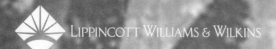

LIPPINCOTT WILLIAMS & WILKINS

A5H549ZZ

Plain & Simple Guide to Therapeutic Massage & Bodywork Certification

LAURA ALLEN, NCTMB

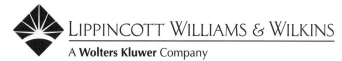

LIPPINCOTT WILLIAMS & WILKINS
A **Wolters Kluwer** Company
Philadelphia • Baltimore • New York • London
Buenos Aires • Hong Kong • Sydney • Tokyo

Executive Editor: Peter Darcy
Managing Editor: Karen Ruppert
Project Editor: Paula C. Williams
Marketing Manager: Christen Murphy
Designer: Risa Clow
Compositor: Maryland Composition, Inc.
Printer: Courier - Westford
Artist: Armen Kojoyian

Library of Congress Cataloging-in-Publication Data

Allen, Laura, NCTMB.
Plain & simple guide to therapeutic massage & bodywork certification / Laura Allen.– 1st ed.
    p. ; cm.
Includes index.
ISBN-13: 978-0-7817-5542-5 (alk. paper)
1. Massage therapy—Study guides. I. Title. II. Title: Plain and simple guide to therapeutic massage and bodywork certification.
[DNLM: 1. Massage—methods—Outlines. WB 18.2 A427p 2006]
RM721.A39 2006
615.8'22–dc22
    2005011736

Dedicated to the memory of
Mattie Bailey Rollins

About the Author

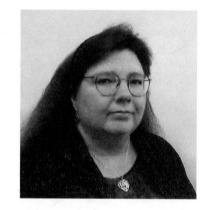

L aura Allen is a nationally certified massage therapist and bodyworker and an approved provider of continuing education under the NCBTMB. She is on the faculty of The Asheville School of Massage and Yoga in Asheville, North Carolina as an instructor of spa therapies. She currently independently offers continuing education classes in Aromatherapy, Reiki, Spa Techniques, Structural Rebalancing, Professional Ethics, and Marketing for Massage Therapists, in addition to teaching the popular class How to Pass the NCE in massage schools and technical colleges all over North and South Carolina. She is a Third Degree Reiki Master Teacher and member of the International Association of Reiki Professionals.

Laura acts as a consultant to massage schools seeking initial licensure, educators seeking approval from the National Board, and therapists who desire to increase their communication and marketing skills in order to effect positive change in their businesses. She also designs and maintains websites for massage professionals.

Laura is a member of AMTA, serves as the Unit Coordinator Administrator for the North Carolina Chapter, and is a frequent contributor to the state chapter newsletter. She is also a member of the Carolina Emergency Response Massage Team that provides massage to emergency responders at natural disaster sites on a volunteer basis.

Born in Savannah, Georgia, to a military family, Laura attended 15 different schools during her family's travels to different military bases. She attended Isothermal Community College to study Social Work, dropping out just short of graduation to enter a career in the restaurant business. Laura owned 4 restaurants over the next 20 years and worked as a chef in some of North Carolina's most prestigious dining establishments. In 1998, she sold her business and returned to school to earn a B.A. in psychology from Shaw University in Asheville, NC. She distinguished herself there by winning the Bronze Award and the Pinnacle Award for academic excellence, and was elected to Psi Chi, the National Honor Society in Psychology.

She graduated from The Whole You School of Massage & Bodywork in Rutherfordton, NC, in 2000, while simultaneously pursuing a graduate degree in psychology through on-line classes. She has completed an additional 120 hours of specialized training in techniques for releasing emotional stress and also completed a counseling internship under the direction of a licensed psychologist, a licensed clinical social worker, and a certified family therapist. Laura remains committed to her own continuing education and frequently attends massage and aromatherapy-related classes.

Laura remained at The Whole You as an instructor and administrator for five years, before leaving to open a private practice that has grown to include seven licensed massage therapists, an acupuncturist, and an RN certified in natural health and microdermabrasion. She is frequently called upon to speak about the clinical use of therapeutic touch and aromatherapy in hospitals, nursing homes, and schools.

Laura Allen is regionally well-known as a musician and songwriter in Western North Carolina and has made numerous public appearances, including being featured on public radio and public television, as well as being a contributor on 3 CDs. She has been a member of the band Hogwild for almost two decades, and enjoys playing guitar, piano, and harmonica professionally as well as for stress relief. Laura resides with her husband Champ, a Reiki Master practitioner and instructor, in Rutherfordton, NC.

Preface

*P*lain & Simple Guide to Therapeutic Massage & Bodywork Certification was written with one goal in mind: to prepare students for the National Certification Examination (NCE) or their particular state's examination.

I was fortunate to have attended a massage school that taught more than 20 modalities and emphasized Eastern philosophy and techniques. Many students aren't as fortunate—blocks of information tested on the NCE often are not covered in their massage schools, leaving them ill-prepared for the exam. This realization, and my interactions with students, led me to write the first edition of *The Plain & Simple Guide,* self-published in 2003 as *The Plain & Simple Guide to Passing the National Certification Exam for Therapeutic Massage and Bodywork.* Although this *Guide* is meant to serve as a review for the NCE, it can also fill in the gaps for those students who may not have been introduced to meridian theory or chakras, for example.

ORGANIZATION

The organization of this book is based primarily on the content areas of the NCE. The book is broken down as follows:

- Part I: Getting Ready for the NCE (Chapters 1 and 2)
- Part II: Anatomy, Physiology, and Pathology by Body Systems (Chapters 3–19)
- Part III: Biomechanics and Kinesiology (Chapter 20)
- Part IV: Traditional Eastern Medicine (Chapters 21–23)
- Part V: Theory, Assessment, and Application (Chapters 24–28)
- Part VI: Professional Standards, Ethics, and Business Practices (Chapters 29 and 30).

The *NCE Study Guide* provides lists of words that the student needs to be able to define; those definitions have been provided here. For continuity's sake, this book deviates from the NCE outline by treating biomechanics and kinesiology as a separate section rather than being part of the anatomy/physiology/pathology/kinesiology section as it appears in the *NCE Study Guide*.

FEATURES

The *Plain & Simple Guide to Therapeutic Massage & Bodywork Certification* has a number of features that make it fun and interesting to read—something that is lacking in the review guides that just list questions and answers. These features include:

- **Inspirational quote** about learning and test-taking begins each chapter.
- **Important terms** are boldfaced and defined in *plain and simple language*.
- **Basic anatomical illustrations** help the student assimilate the written information.
- **Tips for Passing** in each chapter offer the student great study tips and strategies for taking the exam.
- **Affirmations** in each chapter help the student maintain a positive attitude about passing the exam.
- **Practice Questions** at the end of each chapter test students' comprehension and recall of material.
- An accompanying **CD-ROM** contains three complete practice exams to prepare students for testing, in the format of the NCE.

CLASSROOM TESTED

The *Plain & Simple Guide to Therapeutic Massage & Bodywork Certification* was written in response to students attending my 8-hour preparatory class reporting that their needs were not being met in being prepared to take the NCE. Many felt that their schools were remiss by failing to teach the full range of material that is on the test. Others felt that the existing review guides were insufficient in that all they contained were questions and answers, and lacking in any practical advice on how to study for the test. Some students felt that other guides were too filled with technical explanations and hard to understand.

    The policy in my prep class is that students may repeat at no charge if they fail the exam after attending the class. Very few find the need to repeat, and many report that this *Guide* made all the difference in their passing the test.

SUMMARY

In summary, this review guide provides comprehensive coverage of the content areas of the NCE, presented in a plain and simple manner that every student can understand. Special consideration has been given to including more information on pathology, kinesiology, and Eastern techniques, as students have requested more concentration in those areas during the years that I have been teaching the preparatory class.

    It is my hope for each student that this book is easy to read and that it provides the necessary information for passing the NCE. Good luck!

    Laura Allen, LMBT

Reviewers

William Ashmall, MA, LMT
Director
Onondaga School of Therapeutic Massage
Syracuse, NY

Mary Capozzi, MS, RN, LMT, NCTMB
Therapeutic Massage/Integrated Health Care Program
Finger Lakes Community College
Canandaigua, NY

Cindy E. Farrar, NCMT
Assistant Director of Education
Integrated Massage & Deep Tissue Therapy Program
Atlanta School of Massage
Atlanta, GA

Ardath Lunbeck, MS Zoology and Physiology
Sheridan College
Sheridan, WI

William J. Ryan, PhD., RN
Associate Professor
Exercise and Rehabilitative Sciences Department
Slippery Rock University of Pennsylvania
Slippery Rock, PA

Ronda S. Villa, LMT
Southeastern School of Neuromuscular and Massage Therapy, Inc.
Charleston, SC

Jean M. Wible, RN, BSN, NCTMB, CHTP
Continuing Education Faculty at Community College of Baltimore County,
Community College of Allegheny College,
Baltimore School of Massage,
Maryland Chapter of the American Massage Therapy Association
Ellicott City, MD

Melissa K. Wollin, AA, LMT
Massage Therapy Program Director
Bryman College
San Bernardino, CA

Acknowledgments

I would like to thank Cheryl Shew, director of The Whole You School of Massage in Rutherfordton, North Carolina, for the education I received there. I would also like to thank the many fine massage therapists and teachers who have had a hand—literally—in my education as a bodyworker: Barbara Benton, Lois Bergman, Phyliss Velez, Vicki Bates, Dick Overly, Shala Worsley, Wendy Law, Angie Odom, Larry Green, Sherry Honeycutt, Sandra Tompkins, and Harry Walker. Thanks to Gerry and Janice Parsons for the big push in the right direction at the right time.

Thank you to the wonderful team at Lippincott Williams & Wilkins who have helped a first-time author survive this process without any of us having a nervous breakdown: Pete Darcy, David Payne, Nancy Evans, Karen Ruppert, Kate Staples, and Paula Williams. Thanks to Betsy Dilernia for her editing; although I dreaded seeing all the red ink, the book is much better for it. Thanks to Mary McClurkin, who has spent years trying to turn me into a better writer. Thanks to the reviewers, who not only caught my technical mistakes, but provided encouraging words along with their corrections.

Thanks to my mother, Margaret Lawson, for always thinking I can do anything I want to. And my profound and lasting love and gratitude to my husband and rock, Champ Allen, for supporting me in every endeavor I have ever undertaken.

Contents

PART 1

Getting Ready for the NCE

CHAPTER 1

A Positive Approach

The secret of getting ahead is getting started. The secret of getting started is breaking your complex overwhelming tasks into small manageable tasks, and then starting on the first one.

—Mark Twain

Few things in life seem as daunting to the potential massage therapist as the National Certification Examination (NCE). You have invested the money and time to go to school, have performed a couple of hundred practice massages by now, passed the final examination, received your diploma, and now the time has come to get down to the business of what you want to become: a licensed massage therapist. The final qualifying step is passing the NCE, or the particular examination your state may require. Many state examinations are similar to or based on the NCE. For some, this final step simply means sending in their test application on the day they graduate, appearing at the test center with no more stress than a trip to the grocery store, and having their license in hand approximately 1 month later. Others may find preparing for and taking the NCE to be stressful experiences.

I have seen lots of students who graduated from massage school a year ago (or much longer) who still have not gone to take the test. Their reasons vary: "I haven't had the time," "As soon as the kids are in school," "I just haven't gotten around to studying yet." Whatever the excuse, it often boils down to one thing: test anxiety. I know former students who are great therapists, who have the skill and knowledge to teach a class and talk intelligently about the subject at hand, be it anatomy or neuromuscular therapy, but say the word "test" to them and you instantly get that "deer in the headlights" look. Maybe the person with that look is you.

LETTING GO OF STRESS

The key to passing the NCE is letting go of the anxiety associated with any examination. If you follow these simple steps, you will let go of the stress in spite of yourself. Start by taking a deep breath and letting it go. You have allowed the test to become a looming specter in your psyche, blocking your ability to remember the answer to the simplest of questions that you could answer immediately if you were sitting in class. Right this minute, before you read another word of this book, take a deep breath and let it go.

Begin immediately to visualize yourself passing the test. Sit down at your desk or kitchen table. Close your eyes and imagine that you are at the testing center, poised to take the test. Take a deep breath and let it go. See yourself feeling relaxed as you begin the test. Feel yourself relaxing as you begin the test. You are calm. You are confident. You have the knowledge. You are going to pass the test. Take a deep breath and let it go. Practice this scenario several times per day.

Intention is a word with which most of you are probably familiar. You work on the body with intention, so turn that intention inward and work on yourself. If the phrase "I know I'll fail the test" is part of your mental process right now, make a choice at this moment that you are never going to think or say that again. If you expect to fail the test, guess what? You will fail. Thought is very powerful. You will probably find yourself thinking those familiar negative thoughts from time to time. That is okay—you are, after all, only human. But every time you feel a *failure thought* slipping in, take a deep breath and let it go. *Choose* a positive approach. Choose a mantra, such as "I am passing the test" and repeat it to yourself whenever you feel stress creeping in (Fig. 1.1). Use the positive affirmations at the end of the chapters every day. A positive attitude is half the battle in any situation—and that goes double for taking tests!

To a large extent, we choose our own forms of stress. Of course, life-threatening

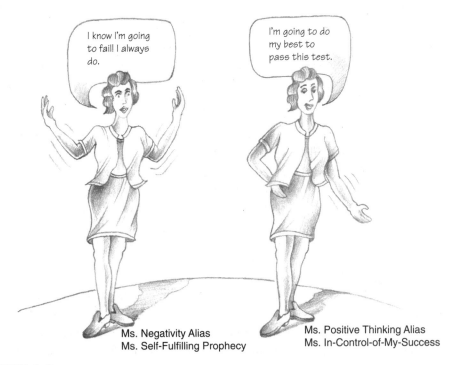

FIGURE 1.1
The power of positive thinking.

situations, such as illness, and life-changing events, such as a death in the family, are stressful for anyone. However, a lot of the stress we experience daily is stress that we choose to have, and sometimes it is not even our own to claim. We stress over what our neighbors and friends are doing. We stress over not having enough, even when our every need is being met. We stress over things we have no control over, like whether it will rain on our vacation or whether there will be a nuclear war. *Choosing to not worry about those things is an incredibly liberating experience.* If you do not waste time stressing over things you cannot control, you will have a lot more time to focus on the things you really want, such as creating a successful massage practice.

Here is a good rule of thumb for letting stress take over: ask yourself if the stressor is going to make a difference in your life a year from now. If it is, go ahead and get angry, wallow in self-pity, or do whatever you have to do to make yourself feel better about it. However, if the stressor is going to be over tomorrow or next week, why waste your energy on it? Take a deep breath and let it go.

Using Defusion

A technique that can be helpful is called emotional stress defusion. Defusion works on the principle that our negative reactions in the present are caused by stress that we had during a past experience. Stop and think for a minute. Imagine you are still a senior in high school, and just watch the years roll back like scenes in a film. Imagine you are 15, 14, 13, all the way back to age 6 in the first grade. Were you scared or excited your first day of school? Did you do well in school and have fun there, or are your memories of getting in trouble? Was there a teacher who made you feel bad about yourself? Did someone call you dumb? This is just a short glance into the psyche, not a long psychoanalysis. Place one hand across your forehead and one at the back of the head. Close your eyes and see yourself at school. If you did poorly or had stress there for some other reason, allow yourself to be there experiencing the same disappointment, stress, or grief that you had at that time. If there was a particular teacher, parent, school bully, or other person involved in your misery at that time, imagine that person now. Imagine the person is walking down the road, suitcase in hand, getting farther and farther away. You wish no harm. You only wish for that person to leave your body and the space that person is taking up there. See that person round the curve and go out of sight. Now change the picture. See yourself, smiling, sitting at your desk, no stress, perfectly relaxed and ready to do well on the test. Take a deep breath and let it go, with joy!

Each time you are aware of feeling stress, take a deep breath and let it go. Practicing the defusion technique can be useful for any stressful situation. Here we are applying it to test anxiety. The NCE is not really the monster you have created in your mind. It is simply a test to find out what you have learned in massage school. *You know* that you have learned a lot, and all that information will be up there in your brain just waiting to come out when you take the test.

MANAGING YOUR TIME

Should you study or watch another rerun of *Jaws* on the late show? Should you study or go to the mall with your friends and spend money you really cannot afford on things you really don't need? You will have to make a commitment to yourself that your study time is sacred time and that you are not going to let anything interfere with it unless it is a genuine emergency, and face it—a sale at the mall is not an emergency.

Set manageable goals and a reasonable timeline for yourself. A good way to start is by going ahead and applying to take the examination. Your acceptance letter will probably take a few weeks to arrive. Once you are notified that your application is accepted, you have 90 days to take the test. If you commit to spending an hour per day studying for those 90 days, you should do well.

It is easy to let things interfere with a goal. Whatever you allow to get in your way—will. Are you looking forward to getting out into the world and start making a living as a massage therapist? Are you at least ready to recoup some of the money you spent going to massage school? Prioritize! You can watch *Jaws* again when you have your license in hand.

Prioritizing

If you plan to be a successful massage therapist, recognize *now* that time management will be a vital part of that success. We all have the same 24 hours in a day. Successful time management is all about prioritizing—putting those things that are most important at the top of the list. In fact, a list is a good idea. Some people are list makers and some are not, but the simple act of writing a list of things you have to do and then deciding which of those things is the most important can be a good way to help you prioritize. A former teacher of mine once handed out a blank 1-week calendar divided into 30-minute increments. Our assignment was to keep track of how we spent our time for a week, including sleeping, eating, mundane activities, chores, recreation—everything. When I reviewed my calendar at the end of the week, I sat down and cried—and decided it was time to make some choices. I was a little younger then and involved in many activities: going to school part-time, playing in a drum circle, weekly group meetings, taking a T'ai Chi class and the Healing Touch class that was the start of my massage career, driving around a former boyfriend who had car trouble, trying to keep my house neat and clean—all on top of running a busy restaurant and playing in a band on the weekends.

The irony is that several years before, I had decided I needed more spirituality and less stress in my own life. The T'ai Chi and Healing Touch classes were lowering my stress level and were important enough for me to keep, but some of the other things (including the old boyfriend with no car) had to go! The simple act of keeping that calendar for a week was a big wake-up call for me. In my quest to find more time for spiritual pursuits and self-improvement, I had worked myself right back on to the same treadmill I was trying to get off by making too many commitments and getting involved in too many extracurricular activities.

I also saw how much time I wasted watching television or running downtown to handle errands that were planned in a careless manner, or not planned at all. Of course, if your baby is sick, you may have to make an unplanned trip to the doctor's office. Sometimes the best-laid plans will fall through, but for the most part, how we spend our time comes down to two things: obligation and choice. If you know you have to work every day from 9 AM to 5 PM, that is an obligation. If you have to pick your kids up at school at 3 PM, that is an obligation. The rest is often a matter of choice, and it is up to you to prioritize what is truly important to your goals versus what you can let go of. Now take a deep breath and let it go.

Downtime

When making your priority list, do not forget about downtime. Those who seek massage therapy as a career have a tendency to be caretakers. We enjoy taking care of other people and making them feel good. We will tell our clients that they need to budget their time and money to include regular massage—and then neglect ourselves. Are *you* getting a regular massage? Why not? Call a classmate or two and make arrangements to do regular trades; that way, money is not even a factor. Do you have time for yourself, for your own nurturing and well-being? How can you expect to take care of other people if you do not take care of yourself?

Even 10 minutes per day blocked out of your schedule for meditation can be a tremendous boost to your own wellness. If watching a sitcom and laughing for half an hour is your way of relaxing, do that. Downtime: a walk around the block, playing with the dog, a game of solitaire, a bubble bath—whatever it is that makes you feel refreshed should be near the top of your priority list. While you are focusing on letting go of the stress related to the test, you might as well expand that to other areas of your life. Start your day with a few moments of gratitude and deep breathing. End it the same way.

FOCUSING ON THE PRESENT

The antidote to a stressful situation is action, not reaction. Focusing on the present instead of on past failures is the key. If you have already taken the examination and failed, or had previous stressful experiences with other tests in the past, you are having a stress reaction—reliving the same stress you had before when confronted with the same situation. Forget about past failures, and focus on the present. Do not obsess over the "ifs." Pretend your brain is a television, and change the channel whenever the "what ifs" and "if only" shows come on. This little trick really works. Whatever is causing you stress, close your eyes and visualize it on a television screen, and then just change the channel to whatever you want the situation to be.

Take time for a reality check right now. Think about how your time-management habits might carry over into your massage practice and address them now, starting with your study habits for the NCE. Self-discipline is a necessary component of good study habits *and* running a successful business.

Keeping your focus on the present not only means letting go of past failures but also means not obsessing over future events. Stress on the test is just another stress you do not need, so take a deep breath and let it go. Make up your mind to do the best you can.

A Healthy Perspective

There are many self-help books and methods for dealing with stress. Of course, there are anti-stress drugs on the market too, but it is best to avoid those and stick to holistic methods of stress relief. If none of the methods I have mentioned in this chapter seems to be a good fit for you, try something else. Try thinking of those people who are worse off than you. Yes, you are sitting here stressing about taking a test. What about men and women in combat stressing over whether they will live long enough to come back to their families, or the neighbor whose child is battling cancer? That puts the test in perspective, does it not?

Realize that although it will not do any good to stress about the test, *there is a difference in worrying about the outcome and assuming responsibility for the outcome.* Keep focusing on your goal of passing the examination. Sticking to your study schedule, getting enough rest the night before the test, and practicing your positive thinking skills are examples of embracing responsibility for the outcome without stressing over it.

STRATEGIES FOR STUDYING

If you have never tried studying with another person or even in a group, you may find that a helpful strategy. The students at the school I attended used to form study groups at the beginning of the semester. They would agree to meet at someone's house 1 night per week for a potluck supper—everyone brings a dish to share, along with their books. After the dishes were cleared, they would all sit down to study together. Sometimes it would be a flash-card session; they also made up games like Charades or Jeopardy with anatomy or massage questions. Anatomy and physiology seem less intimidating when you make a game out of learning. In addition to study partners, these groups also provide emotional and other forms of support, such as rotating babysitting, car-pooling, and meal preparation to help each other make the time to study for the test.

If you need extra tutoring to pass the NCE, do not waste time. Arrange it. Perhaps a classmate whom you perceive to be a test-taking whiz, or even one of your instructors, may need some extra money and would be willing to tutor you. I placed an ad in the paper offering tutoring on the examination and got two responses the first day it ran. That experience has evolved into teaching a 1-day class on how to pass the NCE. Your school or another school close by may offer something similar. Take advantage of it.

Another study strategy is to use every practice massage as a study session. As you work on specific muscles, name them to yourself (silently, to avoid disturbing the client). As you go through joint mobilizations, pay attention to the specific muscles involved in the motions. Which one is the agonist? Which one is the antagonist? Which are synergists? These simple acts will help you prepare for the test, not to mention make you a better, more knowledgeable massage therapist.

A SPIRITUAL FOCUS

Many massage therapists view massage as a spiritual practice as well as a physical one. If that applies to you, hold that thought! Ask your Higher Power to help you pass the test. If you have an altar in your home, as I do, place your intention of passing the test on it. You will find that *focusing* will serve you well. If you are not naturally prone to being a focused person, make up your mind that you are going to be one until you pass the test.

A FEW FACTS ABOUT THE NCE

- It is a pass/fail test. If you can answer 70% of the questions correctly, you will pass. No one (except you) should expect to get 100%. Passing by 70% will earn you national certification. Saying this is not intended to discourage those who are capable of it from achieving a higher grade, but there is no prize for it, either.
- According to the NCE Study Guide, there are 170 questions on the test, but 20 of those are being "pre-tested" for validity, reliability, etc. You are actually graded on 150 questions.
- The test is administered in a nice, quiet room.
- You have 3 hours to complete the test.
- The test is given on a touch-screen computer. The test administrator will come into the room with you to give you a thorough demonstration before you begin.

- You can save the questions you do not know the answer to and go back to them later, and that should be your strategy. Answer all the ones you know off the top of your head, and save the rest. Then go back to them at the end and read them carefully.
- If you have a learning disability or handicap that would warrant it, you may request an oral test.
- It is nearly impossible to cheat. The NCE is a *floating* test, meaning there is a huge computer database of questions, and the computer will pick yours at random. You will not be taking the same test as the person beside you; the person who takes it after you will receive a different test.
- The test is in multiple-choice format. Many times you can read the answers and toss out two of them automatically, or recognize the correct answer when you see it written in front of you.
- There is no waiting for the results. You will find out immediately whether you passed or failed.
- In the *highly unlikely* event that you do not pass, you are allowed to take the test again (and of course you must pay the fee each time you take it).

Do Not Get Discouraged

In the event that you fail your test, the score report will reflect your weak content areas. Do not beat yourself up. It is tough not to fall into the "I am a failure" mode of thinking, but do not do it. Give yourself a few days to regroup, and immediately reapply to take the examination. Do not allow a failure to obstruct your timeline and the goals you have set for yourself. Putting it off for a long period of time is not going to benefit you at all. Although it may seem like a struggle to get right back on the horse that threw you off, that is the right thing to do.

Remember that failing the test does *not* mean you are not a good therapist. It means you need to study more in the content areas that are not your strongest. As soon as you resume studying, focus on those areas. If you did really well in the theory and practice part of the test, do not spend much time reviewing those subjects. Focus on the areas you did not know. Failing may also mean you were just too nervous to do well, and this is where the positive thinking, affirmations, and study tips in this guide can help you.

 Tips for Passing

Keep the calendar (mentioned earlier) for a week, and see how your time is actually being spent. Then schedule your study time as if it is an obligation. Do not try to schedule more than an hour per day. Some people may only have a half-hour or 15 minutes per day to study. The point is, schedule it and make that written in stone. Remember, whatever *you allow* to get in your way will get in your way.

Affirmation

I am in control of my schedule. I have all the time I need.

CHAPTER 2

Coverage on the Test

As long as learning is connected with earning, as long as certain jobs can only be reached through examinations, so long must we take this examination system seriously.

—E. M. FORSTER

TEST CONTENT

The National Certification Board for Therapeutic Massage and Bodywork (NCBTMB) makes it fairly easy to study for the examination by telling you what's on it. Although they don't tell you the specific questions, they do tell you exactly what subject areas you need to study and how the subjects are weighted. The NCBTMB is in the process of implementing a new entry-level certification in massage and revising the existing certification in massage therapy and bodywork; these tests will be replacing the older version in July 2005.

According to guidelines for the new massage-only certification, general knowledge of body systems, including anatomy, physiology, and pathology, make up 14% of the test; detailed knowledge of anatomy, physiology, and kinesiology make up 26% of the test; 14% pertains to pathology; 16% covers therapeutic massage assessment; 24% covers massage theory and applications; and professional standards, ethics, and business practices make up the remaining 6%. The revised version of the examination for certification in massage therapy and bodywork is weighted in the following manner: general knowledge of body systems, including anatomy, physiology, and pathology make up 16% of the test; detailed knowledge of anatomy, physiology, and kinesiology make up 26% of the test; 12% pertains to pathology; 18% covers therapeutic massage assessment; 22% covers massage theory and applications; and professional standards, ethics, and business practices make up the remaining 6%.

In my experience, anatomy, physiology, kinesiology, and pathology are the areas that most students need to apply the most efforts toward learning. Many of the professional standards, ethics, and business practice questions can be answered by using common sense. One advantage some students have over others is that some massage schools are now including the study of Eastern philosophy and modalities in their curriculums. Many schools still teach only Swedish massage and/or neuromuscular therapy. If that's the case at your school, it's important for you to equip yourself with some basic knowledge of Eastern theories and practices, unless you intend to take the newer massage-only certification examination.

The massage and bodywork examination has questions pertaining to many modalities. No matter how comprehensive your school, no school teaches everything. Because it's impossible for you to know everything, take a deep breath and let it go.

THREE COGNITIVE LEVELS

Whether you are taking the NCE or a state examination, the intent of the test is to measure your level of competency and to ascertain whether you possess the knowledge to perform bodywork in a manner that is safe and effective for the client. The anatomy, physiology, kinesiology, and pathology are the scientific parts of the NCE that are consistent with learning objectives for the entry-level massage practitioner.

According to the *NCE Candidate Handbook,* there are three cognitive levels, or learning categories, that form the basis of the questions. Level 1 questions test factual recall and comprehension of scientific facts. This is where memorization and repetition are most important. You are expected to commit to memory scientific data about the structure and function of the human body and related pathologies. Answers are right or wrong; there are no gray areas or "maybes." Examples of Level 1 questions are: "What is the correct name for the collarbone?" "What is the supine position?" There is only one name for the collarbone: clavicle. There is only one way to be supine: face up. (Remember that by visualizing being face up, you can see the pine trees.) Memorization is the only way to answer Level 1 questions.

Level 2 questions test identification and application. The questions require the use of recall and reasoning in the understanding of concepts and how they apply to the practice of bodywork and massage. Definitions, terminology, rules, laws, and standards of practice fall under this category of learning. Again, memorization is the key to passing this part of the test. An example of a Level 2 question would be: "What is the relationship between tsubos and meridians?" This type of question assumes you have studied Eastern theory, that you have an intelligent picture in your mind of the meridians and the tsubos, and that you can relate one to the other. A meridian is basically a line of tsubos that are connected electrically. If you recall that meridians are the electrical pathways of the body, thinking of the tsubos as circuit breakers may help you out. Sometimes forming a mental picture is a big aid in answering questions that appear abstract on the surface.

Level 3 questions test synthesizing and problem solving. These questions require you to analyze information and make appropriate decisions based on logic. These are often the most difficult questions, because they require you to recognize terminology and information and logically apply them through reasoning. Level 3 questions incorporate the knowledge that is measured in Level 1 and Level 2 questions, and they require you to apply that knowledge to a decision-making process. An example of a Level 3 question might be: "A client who has been referred for several visits by a physician for stress and muscle tension seems uncomfortable on the first visit and unsure that about even wanting a massage. The client never fully relaxed during the first session, and when the client returned for the second session, you notice hives had broken out. What is the best course of action?" Level 3 questions require critical thinking. It may seem to you that more than one answer would fit. Choose the one you think is best, and don't try to second-guess yourself.

Suppose the choices for the above scenario were as follows:

a. Send the client home without rescheduling.

b. Give the client a massage anyway.

c. Give the client a stern talking-to about being uncooperative.

d. Call the client's physician.

Which one are you going to choose? Calling the physician is the correct answer. Why? The primary consideration is that the doctor had sent the client to a massage therapist in the first place, so choice *a* does not seem appropriate. The client has hives, and hives are a contraindication for massage, so that eliminates choice *b*. A sure way to make a bad impression, not to mention overstepping boundaries, is by accusing the client of being uncooperative (even if it is true), so that leaves out choice *c*. The right thing to do is that mentioned in choice *d*, call the physician.

TEST FORMAT

The NCE consists exclusively of multiple-choice questions. Even if that might not be the format of the test in states that have their own examination instead of the NCE, using multiple-choice for studying will still be beneficial. All of the questions on the NCE have four choices. According to the *Candidate Handbook,* there are no "trick" questions; all choices are *plausible,* but only one is correct. The other three choices are referred to as "distractors;" they distract you from the right answer. Your strategy should be to read the question carefully, then read all the answers before choosing the best one. Some of the practice questions in this book contain an element of humor, something you will not see on your actual examination. I have included humor as comic relief—a little laugh to break the stress cycle and make you stop holding your breath.

PREPARING FOR THE TEST

Some states may include a practical part on their examination. That was the case in my state (North Carolina) many years ago when the American Massage Therapy Association (AMTA) administered the only test a potential therapist could take for certification or credibility; licensure did not yet exist. A practical examination may require that you demonstrate proper draping techniques, demonstrate conducting a pre-session client history interview, and/or giving a massage in the presence of the examination proctors, who are usually experienced therapists who have volunteered to administer examinations. The NCE does not currently require a practical component on the examination.

Something to consider is that the NCE and most state examinations are created by massage therapists—professionals who are already working in the field. Questions are scrutinized for validity, appropriate content, and clarity before being added to the test. Moreover, questions are "tested" on the test; although they may appear on your test, questions that have not yet been proven to be timely or appropriate are not included in the scoring process until they have been carefully validated.

No single book or study guide is going to tell you everything you need to know to pass your examination. The National Board recommends using two different books in each of the major subject areas for differing perspectives. Doing so can be tricky, especially if the books disagree in any area. For example, some textbooks treat cancer as a definite contraindication, and yet the wonderful book *Medicine Hands* by Gayle MacDonald is all about massaging people with cancer. I repeat the importance of studying your anatomy textbook and your massage theory book. Try answering the end-of-chapter questions and taking the tests in the books. Some of those questions may require writing answers in essay form. Although you will not be writing essay-type answers on the NCE, it will still be good practice, especially for the Level 3 questions. Doing so will make you more familiar with the logical deduction process that is ultimately necessary for passing the examination.

You will also want to use other books and resources besides your textbooks. *Touch for Health* by John Thie, DC, is one of the best books on easy-to-understand explanations of the meridians. *Anatomy of Movement* by Blandine Calais-Germain is beautiful in its simplicity in explaining and illustrating the body's structure and functions. The Internet has made the whole world of research and study available; medical schools and colleges have web sites that are often accessible to the public, and they are a good resource for lessons in anatomy and practice tests. If your school did not focus on Eastern philosophy and techniques, the Internet is a useful resource for studying those subjects as well.

Massage schools vary widely in the amount of testing required of the students. At the school I attended, we had only one big final examination, preceded by a couple of take-home, open-book tests. Other schools test every week. Whichever is the case at your school, save those tests. They are good study tools.

TERMINOLOGY

Crucial to your preparation for the test is making sure you have a thorough understanding of terminology. Again, memorization is the key. By committing the most common prefixes, roots, and suffixes to memory, you will be able to decipher most terms you'll encounter on the NCE. According to the *NCE Study Guide,* in addition to medical terminology, you should also familiarize yourself with the terminology of research, the terminology of health and pathology, and the terminology of position and location. In addition, the field of massage and bodywork has terminology of its own, as do the subjects of professional ethics and business practices.

The general terminology of health and pathology is discussed in Chapter 3; pathology terms relating to each body system are defined in the body system chapters. The terminology of position and location should already be committed to memory. You probably already know what distal, proximal, and sagittal mean, but if you're unsure, learn those terms now before you proceed any further. The structures and functions of the body and its systems are a major part of the NCE, and you cannot hope to understand them or answer the questions if you don't know the terminology first. According to the *NCE Study Guide,* even the terms they have provided cannot cover all the information that might be needed to answer the examination questions. The responsibility is on you to seek all the information and help you can get.

ANATOMY, PHYSIOLOGY, AND KINESIOLOGY

As mentioned, much of the NCE focuses on anatomy, physiology, and kinesiology. This content area is reviewed in parts II and III of this guide. For ease of reference, this guide deviates from the NCE outline in that kinesiology and biomechanics are given their own section (part III). These questions include the organization of body structure from the chemical level through all the major systems, all their components, their locations, and their functions. Massage is about more than muscles. All the body systems—skeletal, muscular, nervous, cardiovascular, lymphatic, digestive, respiratory, urinary, integumentary, endocrine, and reproductive—are covered on the examination.

This section of the test also includes the craniosacral system, which the National Board recognizes as a separate system; some Western forms of medicine do not. If your particular school skipped the craniosacral system, you may want to obtain a copy of *Your Inner Physician and You* by John Upledger for a relatively simple explanation. Eastern theories and techniques are included in this section of the examination. Meridian theory, the five-element theory, and other energetic systems are included in this part of the examination as well. Traditional Eastern medicine is discussed in part IV of this guide.

I remember my surprise at being confronted with questions about the chakras when I took the NCE. Because my focus as a therapist is largely on energy work, I was pleased—but still surprised. Basic principles of biomechanics and kinesiology, including safe and efficient movement patterns and proprioception, are covered in this part of the test as well.

PATHOLOGY

Twelve to fourteen percent of the NCE focuses on pathology and the recognition of various conditions, depending on which version of the examination you are taking. This content area is reviewed in part II of this guide. Emotional states and how stress contributes to disease or dysfunction, how abuse or trauma relates to disease, how the client's medical history affects injury recovery, and the effects of life stages on basic health and well-being are all covered in this part of the examination. Signs and symptoms of the various pathologies, as well as understanding the physiological and emotional changes they may cause, are crucial, as is an understanding of the body's own healing mechanisms. This doesn't mean you are going to diagnose anything, but if you are unable to recognize shingles, you might not realize they are a contraindication for massage. During the intake process, clients should inform you of all conditions that are affecting them at the time or in the recent past. An educated therapist is one who knows when to massage and when not to, and to call the doctor if there is any doubt. It is always better to err on the side of caution. Many of the most common pathological conditions are defined in this guide. This is scientific information you have to commit to memory.

MASSAGE AND BODYWORK THEORY AND ASSESSMENT

Forty percent of the NCE pertains to the combined theory, assessment, and application of massage and bodywork. This section of the test includes general questions as well as more specific questions pertaining to the different modalities. This content area is reviewed in part V of this guide. Because it is impossible to know every modality, take a deep breath and let that go right now. This guide includes brief descriptions of most of the well-known modalities. It also mentions some of the practitioners who developed the methods. Although some modalities (Eastern, in particular) have their own assessment techniques, there are general rules for assessment: analyzing the client's gait and/or posture (Fig. 2.1), taking a thorough health history and interviewing the client, palpation, range of motion exercises, and so on.

The NCE has questions about practitioner awareness—the effects of touch on clients; your own awareness during a session, including the correct use of body mechanics; and teaching your client to use corrective exercises and practice good body mechanics. The effects of gravity on the body and the integration of anatomy and physiology are included in the questions on assessment.

The application questions will address contraindications, universal precautions, and proper draping procedures. On a deeper level, the physiological and emotional effects of touch on the client and the therapist's appropriate responses to a client's emotional states through the effective use of verbal and nonverbal communication are included. Questions about various methods and the effects of hydrotherapy appear in this section of the test, as do questions about CPR and basic first aid.

Principles of holistic health are found in this section of the examination. The word "holistic" (or "wholistic") means relating to a connection among all aspects of a problem, concern, or issue. In the massage industry, holistic is analogous to body/mind/spirit, the idea that disease in one aspect means disease in all: that physical maladies are merely symptomatic of unresolved emotional and spiritual issues. "Holistic" has

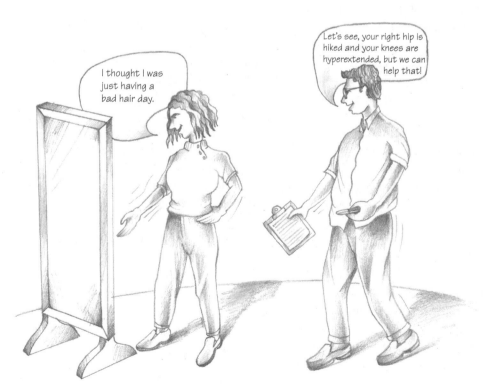

FIGURE 2.1
Postural analysis.

also become synonymous with "natural" in reference to treatments and lifestyles. Massage is a holistic treatment in many ways.

General questions regarding stress relief and relaxation techniques also are found in this section of the test. In addition to massage and bodywork, these holistic techniques might involve aromatherapy, autogenic exercises, meditation, T'ai Chi, and more. Holistic can also refer to education—a well-rounded one. If your massage school did not address some of the content areas, it is your responsibility to study them on your own or to get help wherever you can. For instance, some schools still won't mention the word "energy." There are schools (and students) who think Reiki or a belief in the meridians or Healing Touch goes against their religious beliefs because these systems come from the East. After you pass the test, if you never want to think about Reiki or other energy work again, don't, but it is on the test, unless you are taking the massage-only certification. Just because you have to read something and study it to pass a test does not mean you have to adopt it for your personal belief system.

Basic principles of nutrition are also covered in this section of the test. Most information about nutrition can be found in the chapter on the digestive system in your anatomy book. Memorize the basics, such as how nutrition supports the body and all its functions, how vitamins and minerals are used, and how certain deficiencies can also have ill effects on the body.

PROFESSIONAL STANDARDS, ETHICS, AND BUSINESS PRACTICES

Six percent of the NCE includes questions on professional standards, ethics, and business practices. This content area is reviewed in part VI of this guide. This section includes client confidentiality and adhering to ethical standards. Questions concern effectively communicating with the client and also with other health care professionals. Establishing a relationship with other health care professionals enhances your practice and theirs, not to mention benefits the client. Doctors, chiropractors, naturopaths, nurse practitioners, and midwives are all potential sources of mutual referrals. Professional communications with other health care practitioners, proper record-keeping and income-reporting procedures, basic business and accounting practices, and maintaining safe, legal, and ethical procedures for a massage practice are covered in this content area. Whereas standards of practice and ethical codes may vary from state to state, the material in this guide is a good indication of what is expected of a professional, ethical bodyworker and representative of what would be covered on most state examinations.

Ethics questions on the test may include "fire drills"—examples of tricky situations in which we may find ourselves—and choosing the correct answer will affirm that you know how to act properly in a potentially ethical dilemma. You are just beginning your career as a therapist and haven't had time yet to be confronted with many problems. Studying the sections on ethics in your textbooks and rereading the Code of Ethics as set forth by the National Board, the AMTA, or your state or local organization will prepare you to not only answer the questions on the examination but also respond appropriately when some situation takes you by surprise. No one goes to work expecting a question of ethics to arise, but by the mere nature of what we do—placing our hands on unclothed people—we should be prepared in case something does happen.

PROFESSIONAL CREDIBILITY

Every massage school is different. Although most schools provide a curriculum to prepare students for passing the NCE, that is not always the case. If you live in a state with no licensure requirements, you may not need to take any test at all—and that may be all the more reason for you to take it. In areas where massage and bodywork have not yet gained the credibility they should have, getting yourself nationally certified is a sure way to establish that credibility and set yourself apart from therapists who are not legitimate. In states that don't have licensure, and there are still approximately 20 of them, anyone who wants to can call himself or herself a massage therapist without having any training at all. Passing the NCE is important for establishing yourself as a professional.

 Tips for Passing

Many massage schools have reference libraries with study materials you can check out. Although watching an anatomy video may not be your idea of a big Saturday night, you can probably sit through an hour or two. Make some popcorn and settle in. Sometimes watching a video and seeing/hearing something explained by a different teacher than the one you have at school can be helpful. If the narrator explains something in a slightly different way, it might make sense to you for the first time.

Affirmation

Everything I do turns into success.

PART **2**

Anatomy, Physiology, and Pathology by Body Systems

CHAPTER 3

An Overview of Anatomy, Physiology, and Pathology

Good work is not accomplished in haste.

—Ancient Chinese Proverb

HIGHLIGHTS

Let's begin with some basic definitions. **Anatomy** is the study of the structure of the body. **Physiology** is the study of the functions of the body.

Anatomy has many subdisciplines. **Cytology** is the microscopic study of the structure of cells. **Histology** is the study of tissue. **Developmental anatomy** is the study of the structure from egg to adult form. **Embryology** is the study of structures from the time of fertilization through the eighth week of gestation. **Gross anatomy** refers to structures that can be studied without the aid of a microscope. **Pathological anatomy** is the study of changes in structures caused by disease. **Regional anatomy** is the study of a specific region of the body, such as the head or lower extremities. **Radiographic anatomy** is the study of the body through x-rays. **Surface anatomy** is the study of the body through observation and palpation. **Systemic anatomy** is the study of specific body systems.

The logical order for learning anatomy is to get to know the chemistry of the body, the body's cellular structure, the major systems of the body, their components, their location, and their functions. Massage students left on their own to study may focus on the muscles and bones, ignoring other systems, such as the urinary system or the reproductive system. Don't! Although it might be difficult to see why massage therapists would need to know how the urinary system or the reproductive system functions, it's on the test.

Physiology also has subdisciplines. These subdisciplines include **neurophysiology,** the study of nerves; **cell physiology,** the study of cell function; and **exercise physiology,** the study of the acute responses and long-term adaptations of the body to physical activity or exercise. In the study of any body system, whenever any structure is affected by a pathological condition, the physiology of the structure may be affected as well; therefore, cardiology, endocrinology, and study of other body systems may also cross over into the categories of physiology and pathology. As mentioned, this guide is not meant to be an anatomy text by anyone's standards. For the NCE, you will want to review the anatomy and physiology textbook you had in school.

Another reason to know basic anatomy and physiology is for the benefit of your future clients. Although massage therapists are not allowed to prescribe or diagnose, part of your process is to take a thorough health history of clients before you begin the massage session. The more knowledge you have, the more competent you appear to the client. In my experience, clients often discuss their health problems while they are on the table; some will even ask you questions in the same way they would ask a doctor. Avoid giving unqualified advice. However, if a client asks where the spleen is located or what function it performs, you should be able to answer that question.

Part of your task as a massage therapist is to educate clients within the scope of practice and your own areas of expertise. By offering clients a holistic education that emphasizes the interconnections and integration of theory and practice, you are empowering them and furthering your own goals of creating a successful practice.

Because you have gotten this far in your quest to become a massage therapist, think back to the time before studying any anatomy, and see how much more body awareness you have now than you did before undertaking your massage studies. If you feel a sharp pain somewhere, can you identify its location? Don't diagnose yourself, either; if you're sick, seek help. The point is that it's useful to know where your own gallbladder or Achilles tendon is located. Your own body awareness is vital to your ability to function optimally as a massage therapist. Practicing good body mechanics and ergonomics can extend your career by years. Conversely, working in the wrong way can shorten your career by years! Many therapists have had their careers cut short by hyperextended thumbs, carpal tunnel syndrome, or back pain from working hard instead of working smart.

The NCE includes **kinesiology,** the study of movement, in this content area of the examination. This guide covers kinesiology in Chapter 20.

An Overview of the Human Body

The basic unit of life is the **cell.** Groups of similar cells combine to form **tissue.** Tissue types are defined in their respective sections of the body systems in which they occur. A collection of tissues having a specific function is an **organ.** Organs acting together to perform specific functions are called **organ systems,** which in turn make up the body, also called an **organism.** The organs of the body reside in cavities that are named for the organs or regions in which the organs are housed. The **abdominal cavity** holds the digestive organs and the liver and spleen. The **abdominopelvic cavity** describes both the abdominal cavity below the diaphragm and the **pelvic cavity,** which houses the urinary bladder, the rectum, and the internal reproductive organs. The **thoracic cavity** is protected by the rib cage and contains the vital organs, such as the heart and lungs. The **pericardial cavity** is the specific cavity within the thoracic cavity that protects the heart. The term **ventral cavity** describes the combined thoracic and abdominopelvic cavities. The **cranial cavity,** which houses the brain, and the **spinal cavity,** which houses the spinal cord, together are described as the **dorsal cavity.**

The 11 body systems of the human organism are the **integumentary system,** the **skeletal system,** the **muscular system,** the **nervous system,** the **cardiovascular system,** the **lymphatic system,** the **respiratory system,** the **digestive system,** the **endocrine system,** the **urinary system,** and the **reproductive system.** In addition, the **sensory system** is contained within several of the other systems. The sense of taste, for example, is part of the digestive system and the nervous system; the sense of touch is part of the integumentary system and the nervous system. The **craniosacral system** is often referred to as a separate system, but it is actually part of the nervous system. These systems, as well as the chemistry and cellular structure of the body, are discussed in the chapters that follow. For the NCE, you will be expected to know the organs, the location, and the functions of all the systems, which are summarized in Table 3.1. At the end of each body system chapter, the pathology of that particular system is reviewed.

Directional Terminology

While studying the human body, it is helpful to know directional terminology. The body can be described by planes of division (Fig. 3.1). The **frontal plane** divides the body into anterior and posterior positions. The frontal plane is also called the **coronal plane.** The **sagittal plane** divides the body into left and right sections; the **midsagittal plane** divides the body into equal left and right sections. The **transverse plane,** which divides the body into upper and lower sections, is also called the **horizontal** plane. The body is also described using anatomical directions as points of reference, as listed.

Anatomical position: standing erect, facing forward, arms at side, palms facing forward.

Anterior (ventral): toward the front; in front of.

Caudal (inferior): toward the tail; lower.

Cephalad: toward the head; upper.

Cranial (superior): toward the head.

Deep: far from the surface.

Distal: away from a point of reference; farthest from the trunk.

Dorsal (posterior): toward the back; in back of.

Inferior (caudal): toward the tail; lower.

Lateral: away from the midline of the body.

Medial: toward the midline of the body.

Posterior (dorsal): toward the back; in back of.

Proximal: toward or nearest the trunk or point of reference.

Superficial: near the surface.

Superior (cranial): toward the head.

Ventral (anterior): toward the front; in front of.

PATHOLOGY: THE STUDY OF DISEASE

Disease can be defined as an impairment of health that interferes with the body's ability to function normally. Injuries, poisonings, the introduction of foreign substances, and environmental problems don't strictly fall into the category of disease, but they cause their own pathologies nonetheless.

TABLE 3.1 Body Systems

SYSTEM	COMPONENTS	FUNCTIONS
Integumentary	Skin and associated structures such as hair, nails, sweat glands, and oil glands	Protects body; helps regulate body temperature, waste elimination, production of vitamin D; detects sensations such as hot, cold, pain, etc.
Skeletal	Bones and joints and associated cartilages	Supports and protects body; aids movements, houses cells that give rise to blood cells, stores minerals and fats
Muscular	Skeletal muscle tissue, usually attached to bones	Produces body movements, stabilizes posture, produces body heat
Nervous	Brain, spinal cord, nerves	Regulates body activities through nerve impulses by detecting changes in body's internal and/or external environment and reacting by causing muscle contractions or glandular secretions
Cardiovascular	Blood, heart, blood vessels	Carries oxygen and nutrients to cells and carbon dioxide and other wastes away from cells; helps regulate acidity, temperature, and water content in bodily fluids; blood components aid immunity and repair of damaged blood vessels
Lymphatic	Lymphatic fluid and vessels; also structures that contain lymphocytes (white blood cells), such as spleen, lymph nodes, thymus gland, and tonsils	Protects against disease-causing organisms; returns proteins and other substances to blood and carries lipids from GI tract to blood
Respiratory	Lungs and the airways going into and out of them	Transfers oxygen from inhaled air to the blood and carbon dioxide from blood to exhaled air; helps regulate pH of body fluids; allows vocal cords to produce sound through air flowing out of lungs
Digestive	GI tract, starting at mouth and includes esophagus, stomach, intestines, and ends at anus; also includes organs that aid digestion, such as salivary glands, liver, pancreas, and gallbladder	Absorption of nutrients by physical and chemical breakdown of food and elimination of waste
Endocrine	Cells and glands that produce hormones: pancreas, thyroid, pituitary, adrenal, and pineal glands	Regulates body activities through release of hormones
Urinary	Kidneys, ureters, urinary bladder, and urethra	Produces, stores, and eliminates waste products through urine; regulates blood volume, composition, and mineral balance; aids in red blood cell production
Reproductive	Gonads (testes or ovaries) and associated organs; in females, uterine tubes, uterus, and vagina; in males, epididymis, ductus deferens, prostate gland, and penis	Produces gametes in gonads for reproduction; regulates reproduction and other processes through release of hormones

As mentioned, each body system chapter contains its own section on pathology. But here we'll review some general terminology associated with disease and injury. Let's start by looking at the roots of the word *pathology*. The suffix *–ology* means the study of, and the prefix *path–* means feeling or suffering, from the Greek *pathos,* meaning disease. There are two main types of pathology. **Anatomic pathology** focuses on the

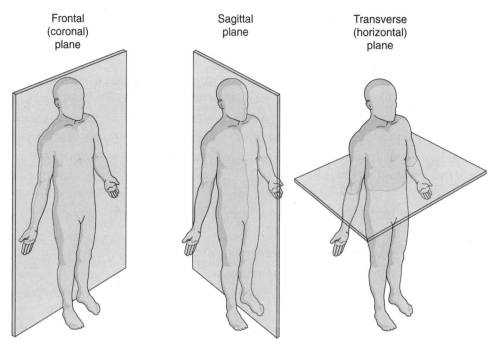

Frontal (coronal) plane Sagittal plane Transverse (horizontal) plane

FIGURE 3.1
Planes of the body. (Reprinted with permission from Cohen BJ, Wood DL. Memmler's The Human Body in Health and Disease, 9th ed. Philadelphia: Lippincott Williams & Wilkins; 2000.)

study of tissues removed from a dead or living person to diagnose disease or cause of death. **Clinical pathology** is actually a number of subdisciplines that are often referred to as laboratory medicine: chemistry, histology, microbiology, and other specialties. To go even further, **pathophysiology** is the study of how disease and/or trauma alters the normal functioning of the body.

To know what is abnormal, you must first know what is normal—not just regarding disease but also regarding simple body function. You may encounter questions on the test pertaining to normal blood pressure, normal body temperature, normal blood pH, and so on.

WHAT YOU NEED TO KNOW

Acute: characterized by sudden onset.

Aerobe: an organism that lives in an oxygen environment.

Ambulatory: able to walk.

Anaerobe: an organism that lives in an oxygen-free environment.

Anaplasia: the irregular structural characteristics of a cell that identify it as a malignant cancer cell.

Anomaly: an abnormal occurrence, especially in reference to birth defects.

Antibiotic: a chemical substance derivable from a mold or bacterium that kills microorganisms and cures infections.

Antibody: a protein produced by the body as part of its defense against foreign bacteria or blood cells.

Antisepsis: the prevention of sepsis by excluding or destroying microorganisms.

Antiseptic: a substance that kills or prohibits the growth of microorganisms.

Asepsis: free from germs.

Atrophy: a wasting away or decrease in size of a cell, tissue, organ, or part of the body caused by lack of nourishment, inactivity, or loss of nerve supply.

Autoimmunity: a situation in which the body produces an immune response against its own organs or tissues, causing severe inflammation and chronic conditions.

Bacteria: microorganisms capable of reproduction; some strains cause infection (and some are beneficial).

Benign: referring to a tumor, or abnormal growth, that is not cancerous and does not invade nearby tissues or spread to other parts of the body.

Chronic: slow developing, recurring.

Degenerative: characterized by diminishing capabilities.

Diagnosis: the identification of disease or trauma.

Disease: an impairment of health that interferes with the body's ability to function normally.

Disinfect: the prevention of sepsis by excluding or destroying microorganisms.

Endemic: characterizing a disease that exists in a location or group of people all the time.

Epidemic: a sudden outbreak of disease in numbers much higher than normal.

Etiology: the study of the cause and origin of disease.

Exacerbation: a marked increase in symptoms or severity of disease.

Fungus: a mold, yeast, or mushroom; some fungi are beneficial; some, such as ringworm and athlete's foot, are not.

Hereditary: genetically passed from parent to child.

Hyperplasia: an increase in the number of cells in an organ or tissue.

Idiopathic: of unknown origin.

Infection: the invasion and growth of microorganisms that may cause cellular injury in tissue.

Inflammation: a protective response from the body in response to infection or injury, characterized by swelling, heat, redness, and pain.

Local: affecting only one part.

Malignant: cancerous; a growth with a tendency to invade and destroy nearby tissue and spread to other parts of the body.

Morbid: diseased or sick.

Morbidity: any departure, subjective or objective, from a state of physiological or psychological well-being.

Neoplasm: an abnormal growth of tissue that may be benign or malignant.

Pandemic: an epidemic that affects an expanded demographic area.

Pathogenesis: the origin and development of disease.

Pathology: the study of disease.

Pathophysiology: the study of how disease and/or trauma alters the normal functioning of the body.

Signs: the evidence of disease as perceived by the doctor.

Sterilize: to destroy bacteria and other microorganisms.

Symptoms: the subjective evidence of disease as perceived by the patient.

Syndrome: a group of signs or symptoms characteristic of a particular disease or abnormal condition.

Systemic: affecting the whole body.

Trauma: a physical injury or wound caused by an external force of violence, which may cause death or permanent disability. Trauma is also used to describe severe emotional or psychological shock or distress.

Virulence: the ability of an organism to cause disease.

Virus: an intracellular parasite that causes disease.

 Tips for Passing

A full-length mirror is one of the most useful reference tools in studying for the examination. Stand in front of the mirror and draw the planes and directions in the air until you have them memorized. As you go through the next chapters, do the same for the bones and muscles. Touch them and say the names out loud several times.

Practice Questions

1. The basic unit of life is the _____ .
   a. Atom
   b. Cell
   c. Molecule
   d. Organelle

2. The study of the structure of the body is called _____ .
   a. Kinesiology
   b. Neurobiology
   c. Pathology
   d. Anatomy

3. *Cephalad* means _____ .
   a. Toward the feet
   b. In the middle of the torso
   c. Toward the head
   d. Toward the pelvis

4. Antibodies are molecules of _____ involved in the immune response of the body.
   a. Carbohydrates
   b. Lipids
   c. Antibiotics
   d. Proteins

5. *Etiology* is the study of _____ .
   a. The cause of disease
   b. The sex organs
   c. Insects
   d. Emotions

Affirmation

I persevere and finish any task that I undertake.

6. The condition characterized by swelling, heat, redness, and pain is known as _____ .
    a. Chicken pox
    b. Fibromyalgia
    c. Cushing's syndrome
    d. Inflammation

7. In the Western anatomical position, the human body is: _____
    a. Standing erect, facing forward, arms at side, palms facing forward
    b. Standing erect, facing forward, arms straight out, palms facing forward
    c. Standing erect, facing forward, arms at side, palms facing backward
    d. Standing erect, facing forward, arms bent at elbow, palms facing up

8. The pericardial cavity is located within the _____ .
    a. Abdominopelvic cavity
    b. Cranial cavity
    c. Spinal cavity
    d. Thoracic cavity

9. The study of the tissues of the body is referred to as _____ .
    a. Histology
    b. Phrenology
    c. Molecular biology
    d. Physiology

10. A short, severe episode is referred to as _____ .
    a. Chronic
    b. Acute
    c. Terminal
    d. Minute

CHAPTER 4

Basic Medical Terminology

Learning is ever in the freshness of its youth, even for the old.

—AGAMEMNON

HIGHLIGHTS

Learning medical terminology may seem like learning a foreign language at first; in fact, Latin and Greek are the main sources of medical terms. You will find medical terminology is easy to decipher if you break the words into their separate parts. Most medical terms have a prefix, a root word, and a suffix. The prefix is normally descriptive of direction, location, amount, or other qualification. The root word is descriptive of the usual meaning of the word. The suffix, placed at the end, alters the meaning of the root word.

THINGS TO REMEMBER

There are several things to keep in mind as you refresh your memory about these terms.

1. Instead of memorizing a whole term, memorize its separate parts. Breaking down a term into its components and memorizing the meaning of the separate parts makes it easier to decipher a term with which you may not previously have been familiar.

2. Think of the terms in their context of the human body. Structure and function are the foundations of understanding the terminology and how it applies to the organism.

3. Watch out for similarities in spelling and/or pronunciation. It would be easy to

choose the wrong answer on the examination if you are confused about the differences, for instance, between the ureters and the urethra.

A good reference book for terminology is *The Language of Medicine*, by Davi-Ellen Chabner, 6th edition (W.B. Saunders, 2001). It's a very comprehensive text. *The Quick and Easy Medical Terminology,* 3rd edition, by Peggy Leonard (W.B. Saunders, 1995) includes terminology in Spanish as well as in English. Both books come with CDs that contain practice exercises.

The *NCE Study Guide* recommends an understanding of the terminology of research. A **theory** is an explanation formulated in an attempt to explain observations in the natural world. A **hypothesis** is a theory that seems to explain a group of phenomena and can be subjected to tests, experimentation, or statistical analysis to prove or disprove. **Research** is a careful, diligent search of relationships between cause and effect, conducted in a scholarly fashion that will hold up to peer review. There are many different experimental designs, from self-report surveys to scientific observation. **Science** is a body of knowledge in a specific discipline or area; the study and collection of data pertaining to a particular body of knowledge through the use of hypothesizing, analysis, theory, models, law, and research is the **scientific method.** At the opposite end of the spectrum is **intuition,** an understanding without the conscious use of reasoning or logic. **Art** is the creation of something beautiful, or the skill to do so.

A **physiological effect** is a change in function. The **body/mind effect** is the belief system that what affects one also affects the other. The **placebo effect** is a scientific term for the power of suggestion—a belief that if something will make you well, it will in fact do so, even if it's a sugar pill, a placebo. "**Somatic effects**" is a collective term for effects on the cells or the physical body (as opposed to the mind or the spirit). Some therapists refer to this as **cellular memory;** the theory is that while you may not consciously remember some past injury or trauma, the body does.

The **general adaptation syndrome** describes the body's short-term and long-term reactions to stress. **Stress** is defined as any factor that moves the body away from **homeostasis,** or balance. Homeostasis is maintained through many **control mechanisms** in the body. Stress sets into motion the general adaptation syndrome, which generally occurs in three stages. Stage 1 is the alarm reaction, the **fight-or-flight response.** Although this response stimulates the body physically, it also causes a lowering of the effectiveness of the immune system, making the body more susceptible to injury or disease. Stage 2 is the resistance phase, when the body adapts to the stress. Stage 3 is exhaustion. At this stage, the body has exhausted itself fighting the stressor. The resistance may be quickly reduced, and the body may succumb to illness because of lowered immunity. **Stress management** refers to our conscious monitoring of stress, developing skills to deal with stress, and the practice of putting those skills into effect.

Some of the terminology on the examination will refer to terms of general health. The terms used to describe the stages of the life cycle are **egg, embryo, baby, child, adolescent, adult,** and **old age. Biological rhythms,** or **biorhythms,** refer to physiological rhythms: temperature, sleep, alertness, and hormone levels. Many of these rhythms operate on a general cycle of 24 hours and are called **circadian rhythms. Ultradian rhythms** help moderate hemispheric dominance in the brain; they oscillate in the minute or hourly range instead of every 24 hours. Humans are also subject to seasonal rhythms. **Entrainment** is the concept that two things with separate rhythms put together will soon adopt one rhythm.

WHAT YOU NEED TO KNOW

As stated earlier, each body system has terminology unique to the system, and these terms are reviewed in the individual chapters. For the NCE, your focus should be learning to recognize and define terminology so you can pass the examination. In the long run, however, proper pronunciation will strengthen your image as a professional health care provider. Therefore, make an attempt to learn to pronounce terms correctly.

I once had an anatomy instructor who was knowledgeable but had some incorrect pronunciation habits. Several times during each class meeting he would give up trying to pronounce the word, saying "you know what I mean." Although I did know what he meant, his careless attitude made me feel a little like I was wasting my money on the class. He was unprofessional and did not last as a teacher.

Certain terms do have more than one pronunciation. If you have Internet access with audio and speakers, there are several audio-enhanced online dictionaries that will actually pronounce words so you can hear them spoken correctly. Your anatomy text is also a source for a more thorough list of terminology and pronunciations. *Taber's Cyclopedic Medical Dictionary*, 19th edition (F.A. Davis, 2001) is a complete reference. Table 4.1 on the next pages lists the most common medical prefixes and suffixes.

Vowel Combinations

- When combining forms are written alone, they usually contain a combining vowel, usually an "o", as in *leuko-. Leukocyte* is one example.
- The combining vowel is used before the suffix begins with a consonant and before another root word. You can drop the combining vowel where the suffix also begins with a vowel, as in *gastritis.*
- Most prefixes end with a vowel and can usually be added to other word parts without any changes.

Pronunciation Tips

- *i* at the end of a word is pronounced long, as in "fungi"
- *ps* is pronounced as an *s*, as in "psychology"
- *pn* is pronounced as an *n*, as in "pneumonia"
- *ch* is often pronounced like *k*, as in "chromosome"
- *ph* is pronounced as *f*, as in "pharmacology"

Surgical Terms

- *-centesis:* a surgical procedure to aspirate or remove excess fluid
- *-ectomy:* removal or cutting out by incision
- *-lysis:* loosening or destroying
- *-pexy:* surgically fixing something to a certain position
- *-plasty:* surgical repair
- *-rrhaphy:* suturing (closing a wound with stitches or staples)
- *-scopy:* visual examination with a light (sometimes invasive, sometimes not)
- *-stomy:* forming an opening
- *-tome:* a cutting instrument
- *-tripsy:* surgical crushing

As a massage therapist, you should be familiar with these terms. Although surgery is not necessarily a contraindication to massage, factors such as healing time, location

TABLE 4.1	Common Medical Prefixes and Suffixes		
Prefix	**Definition**	**Suffix**	**Definition**
a-, an-	without or not	-algia	pain
ab-	away from	-ase	enzyme
ad-	toward	-ectomy	surgical removal
adeno-	gland	-eum	membrane
ambi-	both	-genic	produce, create
angio-	vessel (blood, lymph)	-iatric	specialty
ante-	before, forward	-ism	condition
anti-	against	-itis	inflammation
arthro-	Joint	-sis	process
bi-	double, two	-trophy	growth
brachio-	arm		
brady-	slow		
cardio-	heart		
caud-	tail		
cephal-	head		
chondro-	cartilage		
circum-	around		
cochlea-	shell		
contra-	against, opposite		
derm-	skin		
di-	two		
dia-	across, through, apart		
dis-	separation, away from		
dur-	tough		
dys-	bad, difficult, abnormal		
ecto-	outerede-	swelling	
en-	in, into, withinendo-	inner, inside	
endo-	inner, inside		
epi-	over, on		
ergo-	work		
eryth-	red		
ex-	out, out of, from, away from		

continued

Prefix	Definition	Suffix	Definition
for-	opening		
gastro-	belly, stomach		
glosso-	tongue		
hemi-	half		
hemo-	blood		
hepa-	liver		
histo-	tissue		
homo-	same		
hydro-	water		
hyper-	excessive, too high		
hypo-	under, decreased, less than normal		
ilio- (a)	ilium		
in-	in, into, within, not		
infra-	below		
inter-	between		
intra-	within		
iso-	same		
kine-	movement		
labio-	lips		
later-	side		
leuko-	white		
lipo-	fat		
macro-	big		
mal-	bad		
mater-	mother		
medi-	middle		
mega-	big		
multi-	many		
myo-	muscle		
neo-	new		
nephro-	kidney		

TABLE 4.1 Common Medical Prefixes and Suffixes *(Continued)*

continued

TABLE 4.1	Common Medical Prefixes and Suffixes *(Continued)*		
Prefix	**Definition**	**Suffix**	**Definition**
neuro-	nerve		
ora-	mouth		
orchi-	testes		
osteo-	bone		
oto-	ear		
para-	beside		
per-	by, through		
peri-	around		
poly-	many		
post-	after, behind		
pre-	before, in front of		
pro-	before, in front of		
re-	again		
retro-	backward		
semi-	half		
somato-	body		
steno-	narrow		
sub-	under		
super-	above, over, excess		
supra-	above, over		
syn-	together		
tachy-	fast		
thermo-	heat		
thoraco-	chest		
thrombo-	clot		
trans-	across, over		
tri-	three		
uni-	one		
uria-, uro-	urine		
vaso-	vessel		
viscero-	organ		

of incisions, and the physician's permission need to be considered if surgery has recently been performed on the client.

Additional Terminology

Medicine uses lots of abbreviations and symbols. If you intend to pursue doctor referrals or work in a medical setting, you will benefit from learning medical terminology as well. You may even want to take a class in medical terminology at your local community college. It will be one more tool and will serve you well.

The terminology of biomechanics and kinesiology is discussed in part III of this guide, and terminology relating to Eastern theory is reviewed in part IV. The terminology of bodywork is discussed in part V. The terminology of professional ethics and business practices is reviewed in part VI.

 Tips for Passing

Be alert to grammatical consistency between the question stem and the choices for the correct answer. A choice is almost always wrong if it and the stem do not make a grammatically correct sentence.

Practice Questions

1. The prefix *contra* _____ means
   a. With
   b. Against
   c. Instead of
   d. Behind

2. The prefix *eryth* _____ means
   a. Painful
   b. Out of sync
   c. Red
   d. Bruised

3. The suffix _____ *oma* means
   a. Pimple
   b. Active
   c. Opening
   d. Tumor

4. The prefix *arthro* _____ means
   a. Inflammation
   b. Muscle
   c. Joint
   d. Fascia

5. The prefix *angio* _____ means
   a. Heart
   b. Pump
   c. Vessel
   d. Attack

Affirmation

I have supreme confidence in my own ability in any situation.

6. The prefix *ab* _____ means
   a. Next to
   b. Away from
   c. Inner
   d. Soreness

7. The prefix *macro* _____ means
   a. Little
   b. Big
   c. Death
   d. Bacteria

8. The suffix _____ *ism* means
   a. Condition
   b. Movement
   c. Rate of exchange
   d. Study of

9. The prefix *myo* _____ means
   a. Malignant
   b. Muscle
   c. Movement
   d. Extensive

10. The prefix *nephro* _____ means
    a. Skin color
    b. Bone
    c. Kidney
    d. Sleep

CHAPTER 5

The Chemistry of the Body

Learning is not attained by chance, it must be sought for with ardor and attended to with diligence.

—Abigail Adams

HIGHLIGHTS

Chemistry is not a content area for the NCE. However, understanding the chemical level of the body is the foundation for understanding the functioning of all body systems, so we'll discuss some of the basics. More details about chemistry pertaining to individual body systems are reviewed in the Highlights section of each body system chapter.

An **element** is the simplest component from which all other chemical structures are built. The human body contains 26 chemical elements (not counting the chemicals you might willingly or unwillingly put into your body). Chemical elements are present on land, in the oceans, and in the atmosphere. In fact, 92 elements occur naturally on earth, and another 20 can be created through molecular changes of the chemicals that occur naturally. In addition, there are hundreds of isotopes of the elements that could play a role in the body's functioning (an area of study for research chemists. **Isotopes** are two or more forms of the same atom with different masses.

Chemicals are symbolized using the first one or two letters of their name, usually in English but sometimes in Latin or another language. Oxygen (O), carbon (C), hydrogen (H), and nitrogen (N) account for approximately 96% of the body's mass. An additional 3.9% comes from calcium (Ca), chlorine (Cl), iodine (I), iron (Fe), magnesium (Mg), phosphorous (P), potassium (K), sodium (Na), and sulfur (S). The remaining 0.1% is composed of chemicals known as **trace elements.**

WHAT YOU NEED TO KNOW

Anabolism: a biochemical reaction in which simpler substances are combined to form more complex substances, resulting in the storage of energy, the production of new cellular material, and growth.

Catabolism: a biochemical process involved in the breakdown of organic compounds, usually leading to the production of energy.

Metabolism: the sum of all energy-producing and energy-using processes that occur in the human body.

Body Chemistry and Nutrition

The chemistry of the body is largely dependent on the nutrients taken in. The most important thing we can put into our body is water. Because water is compatible with more substances than any other substance on earth, it is the best transporter for the vitamins, minerals, and other sources of nutrients to the cells. Water facilitates the digestion, circulation, and transportation of nutrients in the bloodstream.

The vitamins and minerals present in food are important to every bodily function, and they must be obtained from our diet because they do not occur naturally in the body (except for vitamin D). Minerals *do* occur naturally in the body, but only in trace amounts, and they too must be replenished through the diet. It is increasingly apparent that minerals play an important role in maintaining homeostasis. The trace elements are aluminum (Al), boron (B), chromium (Cr), cobalt (Co), copper (Cu), fluorine (F), manganese (Mn), molybdenum (Mo), selenium (Se), silicon (Si), tin (Sn), vanadium (V), and zinc (Zn). The role of some of the trace elements is unknown, but they appear to be necessary for the proper growth, development, and functioning of the body.

The body is relatively efficient at regulating its mineral balance. In some cases excess amounts are flushed out of the body as waste, and when reserves are low, more minerals will be absorbed from food, if foods containing the necessary minerals are eaten. It is possible to consume too much of a mineral, resulting in **toxicity,** or poisoning, so it is not wise to consume large amounts of minerals unless prescribed by a doctor. Vitamin toxicity associated with the fat-soluble vitamins (A, D, E, and K) can also occur, but it is much rarer and less harmful to the body than most mineral toxicities. Vitamin toxicity tends to be associated with supplement abuse—the user mistakenly thinking that "more is better," which is not the case.

Chemical elements are composed of **atoms,** as is all matter, living or nonliving. Atoms can be broken down into **subatomic particles**—protons, neutrons, and electrons. Protons and neutrons form the core of the atom, known as the **nucleus.** As their name implies, **protons** have a positive charge, whereas **neutrons** are neutral. Surrounding the nucleus are negatively charged **electrons.** When two or more atoms bond together, the result is a **molecule,** or **compound.** An **ion** is an atom that is positively or negatively charged. Substances that can break apart into two or more ions when placed in water are known as **electrolytes.** Calcium, chloride, iodine, magnesium, potassium, bicarbonate, and sodium are the main electrolytes in the human body. To maintain homeostasis, there is a constant flux in the chemical composition of the body, within certain parameters.

Some substances that form ions when placed into water are classified as either acid or base. **Acids** are substances that will release hydrogen ions in a **solution** (two substances in uneven amounts mixed together). A **base** is a substance that will bind to hydrogen ions in a solution. The gastric juices in the stomach are acid. Other examples of acids are vinegar and citrus juices. Examples of bases are baking soda and bleach. Bases and acids are measured on a scale from 0 to14, known as the **pH scale.** A pH below 7 indicates an acid; a pH more than 7 indicates a base. In a perfect state of balance, the body would be at the slightly basic pH of 7.35 to 7.45. When we put a substance into our body that is at one extreme or the other, we would probably die from the rapid change in pH were it not for the body's buffer systems, which chemically change strong substances into weaker ones. The importance of drinking water and eating a balanced diet are part of a total plan for wellness.

Many dysfunctions or diseases are related to or aggravated by poor nutrition, and some of them can be improved by making dietary changes. Most processed foods contain chemical preservatives and dyes that we simply do not need in our diet. The United States is the most obese nation in the world because of the unhealthy American diet. Poor nutrition and obesity can lead to high blood pressure, diabetes, nutrient deficiencies, and metabolism disorders. It is interesting to note that the U.S. Food and Drug Administration's recommendations of daily nutritional requirements and allowances have changed drastically over the years. The FDA's current Food Guide Pyramid is shown in Figure 5.1.

The process of digestion breaks down food into a more fluid form for nutrient absorption by the body. Food contains the proteins, carbohydrates, fats, vitamins, and minerals that we need to stay healthy. Eating a balanced diet means that you take in nutritionally only what you need for healthy weight maintenance. Excess calories, those that are not burned by the body for fuel, are stored as fat, whether they were initially consumed as proteins, carbohydrates, or fat. Eliminating excess calories will cause weight loss, just as consuming excess calories will cause weight gain.

Proteins are the body's building blocks. Protein is necessary as a source of energy production, although it accounts for only 5% to 10% of our energy, and for the growth of healthy tissue. Protein is consumed in the form of meat, fish, fowl, dairy products, nuts, and grains. Carbohydrates provide the energy the body needs immediately, especially for brain function and many other body functions, such as digestion and absorption. Carbohydrates are found in starchy vegetables, sugars, and grains. Recent research indicates that excess calories in the form of carbohydrates may not be converted to fat as once thought; instead, it appears that these carbohydrates are used for energy production (at the expense of fats). Fats provide stored energy and protect the body and internal organs by acting as insulation, but only a small amount of fat is needed to maintain these functions. Fats are present in dairy products, oil, and some protein sources. Vitamins are necessary for the maintenance of essential body functions and growth; minerals support the structure and help regulate many metabolic processes. If the diet is deficient in any of the necessary nutrients, supplementation may be required to maintain optimal functioning.

PATHOLOGY FROM CHEMICAL IMBALANCES

Pathological conditions throughout the body are frequently related to a chemical imbalance, or chemical "pollution," in the body. **Free radicals** are reactive molecules the body produces as a result of metabolic processes or disease. They are a factor

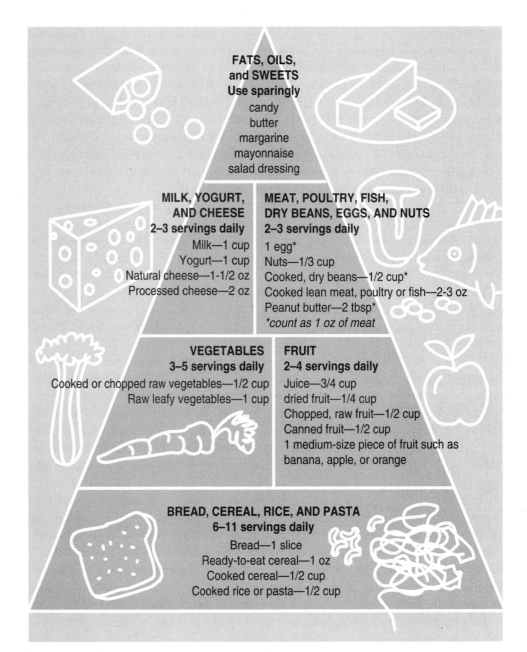

FATS, OILS,
and SWEETS
Use sparingly
candy
butter
margarine
mayonnaise
salad dressing

**MILK, YOGURT,
AND CHEESE
2–3 servings daily**
Milk—1 cup
Yogurt—1 cup
Natural cheese—1-1/2 oz
Processed cheese—2 oz

**MEAT, POULTRY, FISH,
DRY BEANS, EGGS, AND NUTS
2–3 servings daily**
1 egg*
Nuts—1/3 cup
Cooked, dry beans—1/2 cup*
Cooked lean meat, poultry or fish—2-3 oz
Peanut butter—2 tbsp*
count as 1 oz of meat

**VEGETABLES
3–5 servings daily**
Cooked or chopped raw vegetables—1/2 cup
Raw leafy vegetables—1 cup

**FRUIT
2–4 servings daily**
Juice—3/4 cup
dried fruit—1/4 cup
Chopped, raw fruit—1/2 cup
Canned fruit—1/2 cup
1 medium-size piece of fruit such as
banana, apple, or orange

**BREAD, CEREAL, RICE, AND PASTA
6–11 servings daily**
Bread—1 slice
Ready-to-eat cereal—1 oz
Cooked cereal—1/2 cup
Cooked rice or pasta—1/2 cup

FIGURE 5.1
The Food Guide Pyramid. (Adapted from the National Center for Nutrition and
Dietetics, The American Dietetic Association [www.aap.org], and the American
Academy of Family Physicians [www.aafp.org].) NOTE: At press time, the USDA
updated its food guide pyramid. For the most current information on the new food
pyramids and the new guidelines, please visit www.mypyramid.gov.

in tissue damage during the aging process. In addition, free radicals cause tissue
damage from the body's exposure to harmful agents, such as radiation or toxic
chemicals.

Chemical imbalances are involved in many disorders, including clinical depression, diabetes, cancer, and many genetic diseases. Some people are genetically
predisposed to retain certain minerals or vitamins or, conversely, to be unable to
absorb them. The amount of minerals the body absorbs also slows down as we
age.

Tips for Passing

Remember the fourth grade? You had to write your spelling words over and over. You had to write them in a sentence. You had to write the definition. As a result of that exercise, today you can spell. Don't you think the same rules would apply to this situation? Set aside a section in a notebook for words you are having trouble remembering. Write them six times. Write down the definitions. Practice using them in a sentence, such as "A fissure is a crack in the skin."

Practice Questions

1. The body contains _____ chemical elements.
   a. 32
   b. 26
   c. 27
   d. 20

2. _____ is an example of a trace mineral.
   a. Oxygen
   b. Aluminum
   c. Hydrogen
   d. Calcium

3. Electrolytes are substances that _____ .
   a. Are turned into sugar in the pancreas
   b. Break apart into two or more ions when put into water
   c. Are metabolized as fat
   d. Are stored in the spleen

4. When in balance, the body's pH should be within what range? _____
   a. 7.35–7.45
   b. 9.00–9.50
   c. 6.55–6.75
   d. 6.35–6.55

5. Free radicals _____
   a. Help wounds to heal faster
   b. Cause warts
   c. Cause tissue damage
   d. Help blood to clot

6. An ion is an atom that _____ .
   a. Is positively charged
   b. Is negatively charged
   c. Could be either positively or negatively charged
   d. Is neither positively nor negatively charged

7. Chemical imbalances contribute to many conditions, including _____ .
   a. Depression
   b. Diabetes
   c. Cancer
   d. All of the above

Affirmation

I am competent and capable in everything I decide to do.

8. Protons, neutrons, and electrons are all examples of _____ .
   a. Genetic material
   b. Chemicals
   c. Ions
   d. Subatomic particles

9. Excess calories are stored as _____ .
   a. Cholesterol
   b. Free radicals
   c. Carbohydrates
   d. Fat

10. Oxygen, carbon, hydrogen, and nitrogen account for approximately _____ of the body's mass.
    a. 75%
    b. 100%
    c. 89%
    d. 96%

CHAPTER 6

The Cellular Level of the Body

Perseverance, secret of all triumphs.

—VICTOR HUGO

HIGHLIGHTS

The human body and all of its component parts are composed of cells. The **cell** is the smallest membrane-enclosed compartment that can sustain life independent of other entities. More than 200 types of specialized cells perform many different functions in the body. The study of the structure and function of cells is called **cytology.** The study of the function of cells is also known as **cell physiology,** and it follows the process from the time of cell division until cell death. Of the trillions of cells in the body, the largest are no bigger around than a human hair, and the smallest are less than one-tenth that size. Most cells contain three main parts: the plasma membrane, the cyto-plasm, and the nucleus.

The primary function of the **plasma membrane** is to act as a protective barrier and a communicator between the environments inside and outside of the cell. The plasma membrane is **selectively permeable,** which means it regulates what substances may enter or exit the cell. It consists of two layers of fats with proteins embedded in the fat. **Diffusion** is a process during which molecules or ions spread from an area of low concentration to an area of high concentration until the concentration is the same throughout the cell, a state known as **equilibrium.** Diffusion is also called **passive transport** when a substance is diffusing across a semi-permeable membrane. During **active transport,** molecules other than ions are actively transported across cell mem-branes. Insulin is a good example.

The **cytoplasm** consists primarily of a liquid called **cytosol,** which is approxi-mately 75% water; the remainder is dissolved solutes and particles such as ions, fatty acids, amino acids, lipids, proteins, and ATP, as well as waste products. **ATP (adenosine triphosphate)** is an energy source for many metabolic processes. **Organelles** are specialized structures in the cytoplasm that have distinct shapes and perform certain functions, regulated by enzymes. Many organelles act in conjunction with each other. The **mitochondrion** functions in energy production. The **Golgi apparatus,** the **endoplasmic reticulum,** and the **lysosomes** interact to make, secrete, and reduce proteins.

The **nucleus** is a cellular organelle, but because it has so many special functions it is usually considered apart from the other organelles. The nucleus is the most prominent part of a cell and the cell's control center. Although all cells have a nucleus, some cells will lose their nucleus when they mature (e.g., red blood cells). The nucleus contains the genetic material, within **chromosomes.** The **centriole** is a tube-shaped organelle located outside the nucleus. During **cell division** it forms the **spindle,** which ensures that the duplicated chromosomes are equally divided between the daughter cells. Cell division is sometimes referred to as **proliferation.**

A **gene** is a segment of the cell's **DNA (deoxyribonucleic acid),** the genetic instructions that pass from generation to generation (Fig. 6.1). Every cell in the body has more than 50,000 genes, but only a few of them are active at any place in the body at one time, and genes make up only a small percentage of the total DNA. Those genes active in any cell determine the structure and function of tissue and control its metabolism. DNA is a double-stranded molecule that is held together by weak bonds between base pairs of **nucleotides,** which make up nucleic acids. From its location in the nucleus, the DNA controls the synthesis of proteins, which will perform specific chemical reactions. The nucleus also controls cell division.

The human **genome** is the total set of genes in an individual, containing 23 pairs of chromosomes. Every cell has two copies of each gene. Chromosome replication occurs before cellular division. There are two types of cell division: meiosis and mitosis. **Meiosis** is a form of nuclear division in which there are actually two successive divisions without involving any chromosome replication. It results in the formation of four daughter cells, each of which is **haploid,** meaning it possesses a single set of unpaired chromosomes. The union of an egg and sperm during fertilization yields a **diploid** egg, with a full set of paired chromosomes.

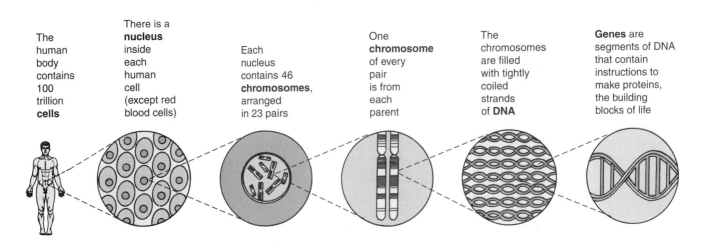

The human body contains 100 trillion **cells**

There is a **nucleus** inside each human cell (except red blood cells)

Each nucleus contains 46 **chromosomes,** arranged in 23 pairs

One **chromosome** of every pair is from each parent

The chromosomes are filled with tightly coiled strands of **DNA**

Genes are segments of DNA that contain instructions to make proteins, the building blocks of life

FIGURE 6.1
Cells, chromosomes, DNA, and genes. (Reprinted from Nettina SM. The Lippincott Manual of Nursing Practice, 7th ed. Baltimore: Lippincott Williams & Wilkins.)

In mitosis, the duplicated chromosomes are separated to give each of the daughter cells an identical set of genetic information. However, during mitosis, errors may occur that result in chromosome anomalies or gene changes. These may cause birth defects or be a predecessor for disease later in life.

RNA (ribonucleic acid) is a nucleic acid that is found in all living cells. RNA aids in the transfer of information from the DNA to the protein-forming system of the cell. One type of RNA acts as a temporary copy of the information of a gene and carries that information from the nucleus to the cytoplasm where protein production occurs. Several other types of RNA are also involved in the protein production process.

Cells are continually working to maintain their homeostasis and therefore that of the body. An understanding of homeostasis has helped scientists develop anti-cancer agents that destroy some cells while leaving others alone, and to create drugs that mimic or block the actions of the body's hormones. As we age, our cells and tissues break down. Age is not so much chronological as it is biological. We expend fewer calories in regenerating and repairing our bodies. We lose lean muscle mass and add fat. Understanding the homeostasis of cells has led to the discovery of many drugs that are designed to control the conditions that accompany aging.

WHAT YOU NEED TO KNOW

Active transport: the energy-requiring movement of ions, nutrients, and molecules across the plasma membrane from an area of low concentration to an area of high concentration, against the substance's concentration gradient.

Apoptosis: the planned death of cells, programmed genetically during different stages of development.

ATP (adenosine triphosphate): a molecule present in all living cells that supplies the energy for many of the body's metabolic processes.

Cell: the smallest, membrane-enclosed compartment that can sustain life independent of other entities.

Cell physiology: the study of the function of cells.

Centriole: an organelle that helps control cell division and the movement of chromosomes.

Channel: a grooved passage composed of proteins that allow substances to flow in and out of the cell.

Chromosome: the thread-like structure found in the nucleus of a cell that contains DNA and proteins. Chromosomes come in pairs, and a normal human cell contains 46 chromosomes (23).

Cilia: tiny hair-like structures that propel single-celled organisms; they serve the purpose of moving particles along a tissue surface, such as the lining of the respiratory tract.

Concentration gradient: an unequal distribution of a substance, often in reference to a higher concentration on one side of the plasma membrane than on the other.

Congenital defect: an abnormality in embryonic or fetal development that is present at birth. Congenital defects may be but are not necessarily inherited.

Cytokinesis: the division of the cytoplasm of a cell following division of the nucleus.

Cytoplasm: the watery substance around the nucleus where most chemical activities of the cell take place.

Cytoskeleton: a network of filaments that provide structural support for a cell and act as channels for some types of cellular transport.

Cytosol: the fluid portion of the cytoplasm.

Degenerative disease: a condition that gradually gets worse over time.

Diffusion: the spontaneous movement of molecules to reach equilibrium, a uniform concentration; occurs naturally and requires no cellular input (passive transport).

Diploid: possessing a full set of paired chromosomes.

DNA (deoxyribonucleic acid): a molecule of the cell where genetic information is encoded.

Dominant inheritance: the inheritance of a trait or disease from a parent who exhibited the trait and had at least one gene for the trait.

Endoplasmic reticulum: a membrane system present throughout the cytoplasm.

Enzyme: a protein that catalyzes biochemical reactions.

Equilibrium: a state of balance achieved when molecules or ions are dispersed evenly throughout a cell.

Eukaryote: a cell that has a nucleus containing genetic material.

Exocytosis: the release of material from a cell by the fusion of a closed membrane shell with a plasma membrane.

Filtration: the passage of liquid through a filter.

Flagella: tiny thread-like extensions that provide locomotion for the cell, are similar to cilia but longer, and in humans are found only on sperm.

Gene: a segment of DNA; the functional unit of a chromosome, which directs the synthesis of proteins.

Genetic engineering: experimental techniques for producing molecules of DNA containing new genes, usually for the purpose of cloning.

Genome: the total set of genes in an individual cell, containing 23 pairs of chromosomes.

Golgi apparatus: a cellular organelle; a stack of membrane sacs where sugar is added to protein and where cellular products are packaged.

Haploid: containing a single set of unpaired chromosomes.

Hydrolysis: the splitting of a compound into fragments by the addition of water.

Lysosome: a tiny sac containing enzymes that digest cellular matter that is damaged or foreign to the body.

Meiosis: a form of nuclear division in which there are actually two successive divisions that result in forming haploid gametes.

Mitosis: cell division resulting in two daughter cells; the process of cell replacement.

Mutation: a change in the genetic material.

Necrosis: the death of cells resulting from injury.

Nucleotide: the basic component of DNA and RNA.

Nucleus: the major organelle of eukaryotic cells; contains the genetic material.

Organelle: a specialized structure within cells that performs a specific function.

Osmosis: the movement of solvent through a semipermeable membrane.

Osmotic pressure: the pressure exerted by water or other solvents flowing into a solution through a membrane.

Phagocyte: a cell that has the ability to ingest and destroy such substances as bacteria and cellular debris.

Pinocytosis: the uptake of fluid material into a cell.

Plasma membrane: the membrane surrounding a cell; it allows the transport of substances into and out of the cell.

Prokaryote: a cell whose genetic material is not contained in a nucleus, such as a bacterium.

Recessive inheritance: the inheritance of a trait or disease when both parents have the same abnormal gene, although they may or may not have the trait or disease; the trait is expressed only when both chromosomes carry the abnormal gene.

Replication: the reproduction of an exact copy.

Ribosome: a cellular organelle; a component of RNA involved in synthesizing proteins.

RNA (ribonucleic acid): a molecule found in all living cells; transfers genetic information from DNA to the cytoplasm.

Selective permeability: the property of the plasma membrane that allows the passage of certain substances into and out of the cell.

CELLULAR PATHOLOGY

Changes in the genetic material (DNA) of the cells can cause inherited diseases and conditions. A single abnormal gene, or abnormalities in the number or structure of chromosomes, can cause birth defects, also known as **congenital defects.** Chromosomal errors, such as the presence of too many or too few chromosomes, occur at the level of the sperm and egg. Each child gets half of its genetic material from its parents. A person can have a genetic disease if the parent who also has the disease passes along an abnormal gene; this is called **dominant inheritance.** Other genetic diseases are inherited when both parents have the same abnormal gene; they may or may not have the actual disease. This is called **recessive inheritance.**

Noninherited forms of disease may also be the result of DNA **mutation.** Genetic mutations may take place in the body over time as a result of environmental factors, such as exposure to toxins. These mutations are not present at birth and will not be passed on to offspring, but they are passed on to all cells in the cell line that develops from the original cell with the genetic mutation. This type of mutation is often thought to be the cause of most cancers. Few cancers are true inherited diseases, which follow the dominant/recessive inheritance patterns. However, some cancers may recur in family members because of a defective gene involved in growth regulation. This inherited gene would be found in every cell of the body; when other cancer risk factors become present in the person's life, that person has an increased risk for cancer.

Degenerative diseases are those that get worse over time, such as degenerative disk disease or degenerative arthritis. As cells mutate or atrophy, the person's condition will deteriorate.

The study of genetics has come a long way in recent years. Today we have DNA testing, genetic mapping, and genetic engineering—techniques that were unavailable a couple of decades ago. Scientists hope that genetic mapping will help find cures for many genetic diseases. By identifying the gene that causes a particular condition, they may be able to disrupt the development of the disease. Genetic testing now allows prospective parents to be tested before conceiving, to find out whether their child would be in danger of inheriting a genetic disease.

Disease results from changes at the cellular level, including hundreds that are genetic anomalies. This list is a sampling of the most widely known conditions:

Amyotrophic lateral sclerosis: a serious neurological disease resulting in the degeneration of the motor neurons; also known as Lou Gehrig's disease.

Grave's disease: an autoimmune disorder that causes hyperthyroidism.

Huntington's disease: a terminal disease characterized by mental and physical deterioration.

Hyperthyroidism: excessive thyroid activity, resulting in insomnia, palpitations, intolerance of heat, and other symptoms.

Hypothyroidism: a deficiency of thyroid activity, resulting in lethargy, decreased metabolism, intolerance of cold, and other symptoms.

Lupus: a systemic autoimmune disease in which the body produces antibodies to its own tissues, resulting in severe inflammation to the vital organs.

Muscular dystrophy: a group of diseases characterized by muscle degeneration when there is no involvement of the nervous system.

Myasthenia gravis: a neurological disease causing a progressive loss of muscle contraction, characterized by a slackening of the musculature of the face and upper body and drooping of the eyelids.

Narcolepsy: a sleep disorder that causes uncontrollable sleep during the day and disturbed sleep at night; may be accompanied by cataplexy, which causes a sudden temporary loss of muscle tone.

Paget's disease: a progressive bone disease resulting in the replacement of normal bone by less strong fibrous and/or unorganized bone tissue.

Raynaud's disease: recurring blood vessel spasms in the digits that causes a pallor (whitening) of the fingers and toes.

Retinitis pigmentosa: hyperactivity of the pigmented cells of the retina, leading to blindness.

Schizophrenia: a group of major psychotic disorders that cause irrational thought, delusions, hallucinations, and bizarre behavior.

Sickle-cell anemia: a disease caused by a gene mutation that affects people of African descent; an inherited recessive condition that causes abnormal hemoglobin in blood cells, leading to infections and organ damage.

Spina bifida: a birth defect in which the vertebral arch does not fuse closed, leaving the spinal cord exposed.

Tay–Sachs disease: a birth defect among people of Eastern European Jewish heritage that causes early death because of the abnormal metabolism of fats; affects the brain and nerves.

Tips for Passing

Read the material! Some schools give out homework assignments; some do not. Even among the schools that do, many times the attitude is, "You are adults, you can read it or not." Many students think if it isn't assigned, they don't have to read it. Get out your anatomy book and look at it right now. Is it well-worn, highlighted, pages turned down, or does it look brand new? If it looks new, guess what—you need to read!

Practice Questions

1. _____ is the study of the structure of cells.
   a. Histology
   b. Cellology
   c. Cellulogy
   d. Cytology
2. Energy for many of the body's processes is supplied by _____ .
   a. ATP
   b. ADP
   c. CAT
   d. DNA
3. The genetic information of cells is encoded in _____ .
   a. DNA
   b. RNA
   c. ATP
   d. ACP
4. Most chemical activities of the cells take place in the _____ .
   a. Spleen
   b. Enzymes
   c. Flagella
   d. Cytoplasm
5. The splitting of a compound into fragments by adding water is called _____ .
   a. Hydrotherapy
   b. Electrolysis
   c. Hydrolysis
   d. Solution
6. Organelles are _____ .
   a. Strands of DNA
   b. Atoms that split as a result of illness
   c. The genes that determine eye color
   d. Special structures in the cell that perform specific functions
7. Mitosis results in _____ .
   a. Two daughter cells
   b. Two son cells
   c. A son and a daughter cell
   d. None of the above
8. Lou Gehrig's disease is also known as _____ .
   a. Multiple sclerosis
   b. Myasthenia gravis

Affirmation

I already possess within me
all I need to become
anything I want to be.

    c. Huntington's chorea

    d. Amyotrophic lateral sclerosis

9. Which of the following affects people of African descent? _____

    a. Parkinson's disease

    b. Tickle-cell anemia

    c. Sickle-cell anemia

    d. Tay–Sachs disease

10. Genetic information is transferred from DNA to the cytoplasm by _____ .

    a. Sperm

    b. ATP

    c. RNA

    d. The Golgi complex

CHAPTER 7

The Integumentary System

I not only use all the brains that I have, but all that I can borrow.
—WOODROW WILSON

HIGHLIGHTS

The word *integument* means "covering." The structures of the integumentary system are the **skin, hair,** and **nails,** along with various glands, muscles, mucus membranes, and nerves. The functions of the integumentary system are to provide protection for the body (think of it as the outer wrap), to regulate body temperature, to provide sensory information, to aid in excretion and absorption, to provide a reservoir for blood, and to aid in the synthesis of vitamin D.

The skin is the largest organ of the human body; in an average adult, it covers approximately 22 square feet. The skin is the most important organ to the sense of **touch. Sensory receptors** are located at the peripheral end of incoming (afferent) nerves. **Pacinian corpuscles** are small oval bodies terminating some of the minute branches of sensory nerves of the skin. **Ruffini endings** are sensory organs located in the subcutaneous connective tissue at the end of the fingers. **Krause end bulbs** are sensory receptors of incoming nerves in the mouth, the eyelids, the skin, and other places that are sensitive to cold.

The skin is composed of two main parts, the epidermis and the dermis (Fig. 7.1). The **epidermis** is the thin, outer layer of the skin. It consists of four strata (layers): the **stratum corneum, stratum lucidum, stratam granulosom,** and **stratum germinativum.** Epidermis is composed of four main types of cells: keratinocytes, melanocytes, Langerhans cells, and Merkel's cells (also called Merkel's disks).

Keratinocytes manufacture **keratin,** the protein that helps protect the skin from such environmental elements as the sun and pollution, and **lammelar granules,** which waterproof the skin. **Melanocytes** produce the **melanin,** which gives the skin color

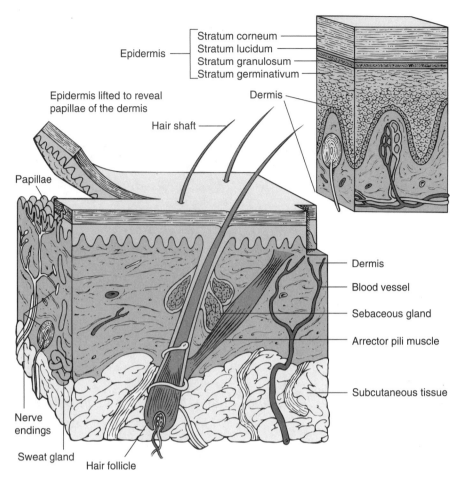

FIGURE 7.1
Components of the skin. (Reprinted with permission from WK Health. Bare BG, Smeltzer SC. Health Assessment in Nursing. Philadelphia: Lippincott-Raven; 1998.)

and protects it against the ultraviolet rays of the sun. **Langerhans cells** are manufactured from the red bone marrow and help protect the skin against microbial infections. **Merkel's cells,** also called tactile cells, function in the sensation of touch. Sensations that are felt through the skin include not only touch but also temperature changes and pain whenever there is tissue trauma or damage.

The deeper, thicker **dermis** is composed of three types of connective tissue. Underneath the dermis is another layer, the **hypodermis,** also called the **subcutaneous layer.** The hypodermis contains **adipose tissue** (fat) and the larger blood vessels that supply the skin.

The thickness and sensitivity of the skin vary according to its place on the body. Thin skin is usually hairy, whereas thick skin is hairless. The so-called thin skin covers the entire body except for the palms, the finger pads, and the soles of the feet, which are covered in thick skin. Thin skin has fewer nerve endings and fewer sweat glands than thick skin. Thin skin has **sebaceous glands,** also called oil glands, whereas thick skin does not.

The primary role of hair is protection. Hair helps protect the scalp from injury and sun damage, and helps maintain body heat. The eyebrows and eyelashes help protect the eyes from foreign particles. Nostril hairs help filter the air we breathe, and hair in the ear canal helps prevent foreign matter from invading the ear. The dead keratinized hairs have two regions, the root and the shaft. The root is the part of the hair that is embedded in the skin. The shaft is the part that sticks out above the skin.

Nails protect the fingers and toes, and also help us grasp small objects. Nails are densely packed keratinized cells. Nails have three regions. The nail body lays on the nail bed, a layer of epithelium. The free edge is the part of the nail that extends past the tissue and it needs to be kept short by massage therapists. The nail root is the part that extends under the skin.

WHAT YOU NEED TO KNOW

Accessory structures: hair and nails; also known as *dermal appendages*.

Apocrine sweat gland: a type of gland that develops along with hair follicles and starts secreting at the onset of puberty. It produces odorless sweat, which supports the growth of bacteria; bacteria in sweat create body odor.

Arrector pili: Fan-like muscles located at the base of hair follicles that contract in response to cold or emotional stimuli; responsible for the appearance of goose bumps.

Carotene: the precursor to vitamin A; each molecule of carotene gives rise to two vitamin A molecules. Too much carotene in the system can give the skin an orange tint.

Collagen: a protein in connective tissue that gives the skin strength and flexibility.

Dermatitis: an inflammation of the skin.

Dermatology: the study of the skin and its conditions and treatment; a medical specialty dealing with diseases and disorders of the skin.

Dermatosis: a disorder of the skin involving lesions or eruptions, in which there is usually no inflammation.

Dermis: the deeper connective tissue layer of the skin; the "thick skin."

Duct gland: a gland in the skin that extracts material from blood to form excretions. Apocrine sweat glands form sweat and sebaceous glands form oil.

Eccrine sweat gland: a coiled tubular gland found all over the body that produces sweat directly onto the skin.

Elastin: a protein in connective tissue that gives skin its elastic properties.

Epidermis: the outermost layer of the skin; the "thin skin."

Free nerve ending: a peripheral end of a sensory nerve with filaments that end freely in the tissue.

Hair follicle: a tube-shaped depression in the dermis; extends to the hypodermis and gives rise to keratinized epidermal cells, or hair.

Hemoglobin: a protein in red blood cells that carries oxygen.

Hypodermis: the deepest (or subcutaneous) layer of the skin; includes areolar and adipose tissue.

Keratin: a tough and fibrous protein; produced by keratinocytes in the epidermis. Keratin in its soft form gives skin its waterproof properties. Hard keratin forms hair and nails.

Krause end bulb: a type of nerve terminal found in the skin, the mouth, and eyelids; sensitive to cold.

Langerhans cell: a type of white blood cell found in the epidermis that helps protect the body from invading bacteria and/or viruses.

Melanin: a brown–black pigment that contributes to the color of skin and absorbs UV rays; produced by melanocytes in the epidermis.

Meissner's corpuscle: a small, oval sensory body found in the papillae of the skin, especially in fingers and toes.

Merkel's cell: a type of epidermal cell that functions in the sensation of touch (tactile sensation).

Pacinian corpuscle: a small oval body found in the terminating ends of some of the tiny branches of sensory nerves of the skin.

Ruffini ending: a sensory organ found in the subcutaneous connective tissue of the fingers.

Stratum: a layer of the epidermis. From most superficial to deep, they are: stratum corneum, stratum lucidum, stratum granulosum, and stratum germinativum.

PATHOLOGY OF THE INTEGUMENTARY SYSTEM

Healthy skin is pliable, slightly moist, soft, and slightly acidic. It is important for a massage therapist to be able to recognize conditions of the skin, to avoid areas affected with conditions that are contraindicated. The therapist should bear in mind that it may also be necessary to refer the client for medical care. Be sensitive, and don't scare your client to death. If you notice a mole, rash, or other skin condition that looks suspect on your client's back (an area that they obviously can't see), you might ask, "Are you aware of this mole? You might want to have your doctor take a look at it." Don't say it looks like cancer. Making a diagnosis is not appropriate for a massage therapist to do. A skin condition that is localized in one area of the body is not a contraindication for massage—except in the affected area.

Therapists should also be conscious of their own skin. Be aware of how it looks to your clients if you have any skin conditions—and definitely do not perform massage if you have a condition that you could pass on to anyone.

The study of the integumentary system and its pathology is known as **dermatology. Skin lesions** occur in a number of different forms, known as primary and secondary. **Primary lesions** are also called **principal lesions. Secondary lesions** develop in the later stages of trauma or disease.

The following are considered primary lesions:

Bulla: a large blister filled with serous fluid, as in dermatitis or second-degree burns.

Macule: a flat, small, discolored area of the skin (e.g., a freckle).

Papule: an elevated, firm, circular area, such as a wart or mole.

Pustule: a small, pus-filled lesion or bump on the skin surface.

Tubercle: a small, rounded nodule, lesion, or prominence attached to bone, mucous membrane, or skin.

Tumor: an abnormal mass of tissue that results from excessive cell division; they may be benign (not cancerous) or malignant (cancerous).

Vesicle: a small fluid-filled blister.

The following are considered secondary lesions:

Crust: the scab that forms on a healing wound.

Fissure: a crack in the skin, such as chapped lips or chapped hands.

Scale: an accumulation of epidermal flakes, such as excessive dandruff.

Scar: fibrous tissue that replaces normal skin after injury.

Ulcer: an open lesion on the skin usually extending to the dermis, the layer below the skin; usually associated with redness, serious moisture, and irritation until scabbing occurs.

Wheal: an itchy, swollen lesion that goes away after a few hours.

Burns are classified according to the depth of the damage. Burns can have serious effects on the body, such as dehydration, infection, or other complications. **First-degree burns** involve only the outer layer of skin (epidermis), which turns red and is painful, such as sunburn. **Second-degree burns** penetrate deeper into the body and may cause blistering. Severe sunburn may also be a second-degree burn; scalding with steam or hot water is another example. **Third-degree burns** are the most serious, involving the full depth of the skin, and might also affect underlying tissues and muscles.

Discoloration of the skin is often related to circulation. **Flushing** is a redness of the skin that may be related to fever or emotional feelings, such as embarrassment **(blushing).** It is usually confined to the face and neck. **Cyanosis** causes the skin to take on a blue tint and is the result of a lack of oxygen in the blood. It is usually caused by heart failure or respiratory problems. **Jaundice** is a yellow discoloration that may be related to blood diseases, inflammation of the liver, or a blockage in the bile duct. **Carotenemia** is a yellowing of the skin that is caused by the excessive intake of carrots or other red or orange vegetables containing carotene. **Pallor,** also referred to as **blanching,** is a paleness of the skin most often caused by a lack of circulation. **Bronzing** is a darkening of the skin that is caused by Addison's disease. **Black and blue marks,** or **hematomas,** are other terms for **bruising.**

Dermatosis simply refers to any skin disease. **Dermatitis** is a skin inflammation that may have any number of causes, such as allergies, chemical sensitivities, or exposure to acids or other toxic substances. **Atopic dermatitis** is also referred to as **eczema,** which is accompanied by intense itching and inflammation. It may include blistering, lesions, and redness.

Other pathological conditions of the skin include the following:

Acne: a disease of the sebaceous glands that may also involve the hair follicles, characterized by inflammatory lesions such as papules and pustules, as well as noninflammatory lesions such as blackheads and whiteheads.

Alopecia: an absence of body hair where hair usually exists.

Angioma: a benign tumor in the skin that is made up of distended blood vessels or lymph vessels that are usually irregularly shaped.

Basal cell carcinoma: the most common form of skin cancer; a malignant growth most often found on fair-skinned people, usually the face, or other areas exposed to the sun.

Blackhead: a small mass of hardened fat and cellular debris that appears most frequently on the face and upper body; an open comedone.

Callus: a thickened area of the keratin layer of the epidermis that results from repeated friction or pressure.

Candidiasis: usually a superficial infection that occurs on the moist areas of the skin, including the mouth, the respiratory tract, or the vagina; caused by the fungus *Candida albicans.*

Cellulitis: an acute bacterial infection of the deep subcutaneous tissue characterized by redness and swelling; may affect the muscle.

Cold sore: an infected sore or blister occurring on the lips or mouth, caused by the herpes simplex virus (type 1). Cold sores tend to appear during times of stress, and infected individuals should avoid contact with others as the infection is contagious.

Comedone: a lesion characterized as open or closed. A blackhead is an open comedone; a whitehead is a closed comedone.

Corn: a keratinized horny layer in the epidermis of the foot.

Dermatophytosis: a superficial fungal infection of the skin, hair, or nails; sometimes refers to ringworm or athlete's foot.

Furuncle: also known as a boil, a growth that results from a staph infection in a hair follicle or sweat gland. A group of boils is termed a carbuncle.

Lice: small parasitic insects that adhere to the skin and cause an itchy, red rash; commonly spread by person-to-person contact. Lice on the body are known as pediculosis capitis; lice on the head, the eggs (nits) of which resemble dandruff, are known as pediculosis corporis; lice on the pubic area are known as pediculosis pubis or crab lice.

Lipoma: a benign clump of fat cells.

Malignant melanoma: a malignant tumor arising from the deep, pigment-producing cells (melanosomes) of the skin; the leading cause of death related to skin lesions. Melanoma is usually irregularly shaped and varies in color.

Mole: a benign pigmented skin lesion.

Neurotrophic ulcer: an ulcer of the neural tissue.

Periungual: referring to the fold of skin surrounding the nails.

Pruritus: extreme itching.

Psoriasis: a chronic, squamous irritation marked by cycles of remission and exacerbation.

Rosacea: a chronic skin disorder of the face caused by inflammation of the cheeks, nose, forehead, and eyelids. Rosacea results in redness and acne-like skin eruptions.

Scabies: a contagious skin irritation caused by the common itch mite, accompanied by tiny eruptions and intensely uncomfortable itching.

Scleroderma: a chronic disorder characterized by hardening and thickening of the skin.

Seborrheic keratosis: a benign lesion caused by excessive growth of the top layer of skin.

Skin tag: a harmless polyp-like growth of epidermis and fibrous tissue growing outward.

Tinea: a general term that refers to ringworm or similar fungal infections; also called dermatophytosis. Tinea corporis is fungus on the scalp; tinea pedis is fungus of the foot; tinea barbae is fungus of the beard/facial hair; and tinea cruris is fungus of the perineum, commonly referred to as jock itch.

Vitiligo: a skin condition characterized by the appearance of irregular white patches, resulting from the loss of pigment-producing cells.

Warts are harmless but unsightly epidermal protrusions; actually, they are small benign tumors. If a single cell becomes infected with the **human papilloma virus (HPV),**

the result is a wart. **Flat warts** occur in groups, usually on the face and hands of children. **Filiform warts** are projected papillae and may number one or many in a group. **Plantar warts** occur on the soles of the feet and are usually very painful. The **common wart** is also known as an **infectious wart.** Warts eventually disappear on their own but sometimes recur.

Tips for Passing

Instead of going on a 48-hour study marathon, set a reasonable time goal for yourself, such as studying 30 minutes per day. Where are you going to find 30 minutes? How about turning off the television? Get up 30 minutes earlier every day, or stay up 30 minutes later. Carry this book with you and read a few lines throughout the day—during your coffee break at work, while you're standing in line at the store, while waiting at the doctor's office, while you're on hold on the telephone, while you're eating lunch. There is so much wasted time in the day. But that's not to say that you shouldn't have time just to stop and smell the roses. In fact, you should definitely take time during the day to clear your mind, take a few deep breaths, and let go of any stress. Carrying a lot of stress will not help you pass the test.

Practice Questions

1. Which of the following conditions could be caused by consuming too much carotine?
   a. Acne
   b. Profuse sweating
   c. Muscle cramps
   d. Orange-tinted appearance of the skin
2. The study of the skin and its pathology is called
   a. Dermatitis
   b. Dermatology
   c. Dermatomes
   d. Oncology
3. The sebaceous glands form
   a. Hormones
   b. Oil
   c. Sweat
   d. Tears
4. The skin aids in the synthesis of
   a. Calcium
   b. Vitamin B
   c. Vitamin D
   d. Potassium
5. Which of the following structures forms perspiration?
   a. Sebaceous glands
   b. Langerhans cells

Affirmation

I am preparing for my career as a successful massage therapist.

    c. Sudiferous glands

    d. Endocrine glands

6. Which of the following is the most superficial layer of skin?

    a. Dermis

    b. Epidermis

    c. Endodermis

    d. Hypodermis

7. A pigment produced in the skin that gives skin color is

    a. Melanin

    b. Keratin

    c. Hemoglobin

    d. Seratonin

8. _____ is caused by a lack of oxygen in the blood.

    a. Addison's disease

    b. Jaundice

    c. Cynanosis

    d. Carotemia

9. *Candida albicans* is a

    a. Bacterium

    b. Microphage

    c. Virus

    d. Fungus

10. Scleroderma is

    a. Skin that has flaked off

    b. Skin that has turned yellow

    c. Skin that has turned blue

    d. Skin that has hardened

CHAPTER **8**

The Skeletal System

Learning is a treasure which accompanies its owner everywhere.
—Ancient Chinese Proverb

HIGHLIGHTS

The study of the skeletal system is known as **osteology.** The branch of surgery concerned with the skeletal system is called **orthopedics.** The structures of the skeletal system are the bones, along with their supporting joints, cartilages, and ligaments. The functions of the skeletal system are to support and give shape to the body, to protect internal organs and tissues, to serve as attachments for muscles, to work in conjunction with muscles to allow movement, to manufacture red blood cells, and to store minerals in the body.

Individual bone cells, or **osteocytes,** are either osteoclasts or osteoblasts. **Osteoclasts** are cells that release stored mineral nutrients from the bones and produce substances that break down bone tissue to remove tissue that isn't needed. **Osteoblasts** perform opposite functions, building bone cells, repairing bone tissue, and storing minerals for future use. The **bone marrow** located within the bones produces more than two million red blood cells each minute to replace those that are worn out and discarded by the liver.

Bones are the hardest structure of the body with the exception of **dentine,** the calcified tissue that surrounds the pulp cavity of a tooth. Bone is both organic and inorganic, containing bone cells, connective tissues, blood vessels, and marrow, as well as minerals. What are the components of bone? Bone cells are embedded in a calcified material, mainly calcium carbonate and calcium phosphate, that surrounds collagen fibers. The hard, dense outer layer of bone is known as **compact bone.** The interior of the bone and the **epiphyses** (ends) of long bones contain a less dense,

59

porous material that contains spaces filled with bone marrow and is referred to as **spongy bone.** The shaft of the long bones is referred to as the **diaphysis.** In addition, long bones have an internal space called the **medullary cavity.** Lining the medullary cavity is a layer of connective tissue, the **endosteum.** Bones have another specialized connective tissue, the **periosteum,** that covers the outer bone surface and acts as a connector to the tendons. Because bone is made of a hard, ceramic-like substance, it is subject to **piezoelectricity,** the production of electrical polarization in the material caused by mechanical stress.

Bones are classified by their different shapes, including long bones, short bones, flat bones, and irregularly shaped bones. The skeleton is divided into two parts: the **axial skeleton,** which includes the skull, the hyoid, the bones of the thorax, and the vertebral column; and the **appendicular skeleton,** which includes the bones of the shoulders, hips, arms, hands, legs, and feet. All together, there are 206 bones in the body; the major ones are shown in Figure 8.1.

Refer to your anatomy book for more detailed drawings. **Long bones** include the humerus and the femur, **short bone** examples are the phalanges; a **flat bone** example would be the scapula, and **irregularly shaped bones** include the hyoid (unusual because it does *not* articulate with any other bone) and the vertebrae. Small bones formed in tendons and irregularly shaped, such as the patella (kneecap), are referred to as **sesamoid bones. Cuboid bones** are roughly cube-shaped, such as the lateral bones of the distal end of the tarsus.

Bones are connected to each other at **articulations,** or **joints.** Joints allow varying degrees of movement and are divided into three classes. **Synarthrotic joints,** like the parts of the skull, are classified as immovable. They are frequently referred to as **fibrous joints. Amphiarthrotic joints,** such as the pubic bones and the sacroiliac, have limited movement. Amphiarthrotic joints are also referred to as **cartilaginous joints. Diarthrotic joints,** also called **synovial joints,** such as the hips or fingers, allow the most amount of motion and are freely movable. Synovial joints contain a cavity filled with **synovial fluid** between the articulating surfaces. These articulating surfaces are called **facets,** and they are shaped to fit together in a manner to allow movement (Fig. 8.2).

The hip and shoulder joints are **ball-and-socket joints.** One surface is roughly spherical and the other is cup-shaped, allowing the joint to move in all directions. The finger metacarpophalangeal joint is a **condyloid-type joint,** which allows flexion and extension, abduction and adduction, and circumduction. The elbow, knee, and ankle are examples of **hinge joints,** in which one surface is convex and the other is concave, allowing them to fit together like a clasp. These joints allow movement in one plane, such as flexion and extension.

The intercarpals and intertarsals are examples of **gliding joints,** where articulating surfaces are both flat and movement is limited. The wrist and the atlas-occipital joint, where the head is attached to the body, are examples of **ellipsoid joints.** An ellipsoid is an oval bone projection that fits into a rough elliptical cavity of another bone. Movement is possible in two planes, flexion/extension and abduction/adduction. The atlantoaxial joint, the joint between the first two cervical vertebrae, is an example of a **pivot joint,** which allows rotation only. A pivot joint is formed by a cone-shaped surface that articulates with a concave surface of another bone.

For movement to occur, bones (and muscles) act as **levers.** The joints function as the **fulcrums** of these levers. Three factors affect how and to what extent a bone is going to move: the position of the fulcrum (joint), the effort required to move, and the resistance encountered. Levers are classified into three different types, according to

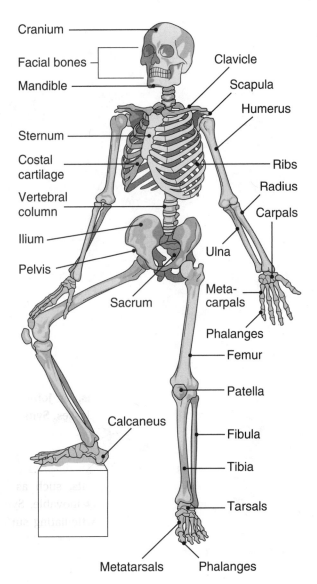

Cranium

Facial bones

Mandible

Clavicle

Scapula

Humerus

Sternum

Costal cartilage

Vertebral column

Ilium

Pelvis

Sacrum

Ribs

Radius

Carpals

Ulna

Meta-carpals

Phalanges

Femur

Patella

Calcaneus

Fibula

Tibia

Tarsals

Metatarsals

Phalanges

FIGURE 8.1
Bones of the skeleton. (Reprinted with permission from
Cohen BJ, Wood DL. Memmler's The Human Body in Health
and Disease, 9th ed. Philadelphia: Lippincott Williams &
Wilkins; 2000. Fig. 19.1.)

these three factors (Fig. 8.3). **First-class levers,** the most rare in the human body, can
be a mechanical advantage or disadvantage, depending on whether the fulcrum is close
to the resistance. The best example is the head as it rests on the vertebral column.
In a **second-class lever,** the resistance is between the fulcrum (joint) and the effort.
Second-class levers are not plentiful in the human body, either. One example is the
ball of the foot, combined with the tarsals and the calf muscles. The most plentiful
levers in the body are **third-class levers,** which include the elbow joint and the adductors of the thighs.

Muscles are connected to the bones by **tendons,** a strong fibrous connective tissue.
A torn tendon will affect the ability of a joint to flex or extend. Bones are connected

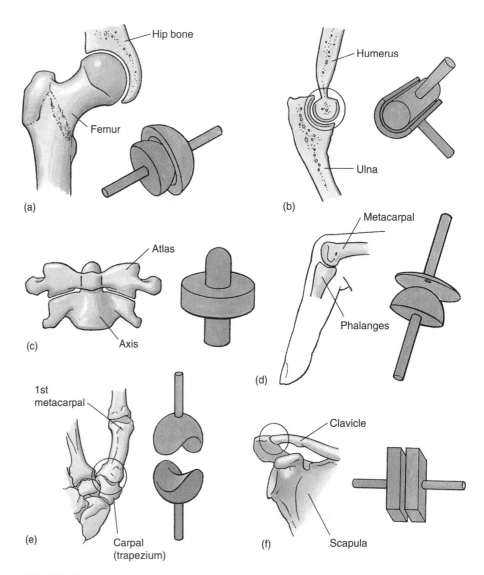

FIGURE 8.2
Types of synovial joints. **(a)** Ball and socket. **(b)** Hinge. **(c)** Pivot. **(d)** Ellipsoidal or condyloid. **(e)** Saddle. **(f)** Gliding or planar. (Reprinted with permission from Moore KL, Agur AMR. Essential Clinical Anatomy, 2nd ed. Baltimore: Lippincott Williams & Wilkins; 1999. Fig. 3.34.)

to other bones at the articulations by **ligaments,** bands of fibrous tissue that strengthen and stabilize the joints.

WHAT YOU NEED TO KNOW

Bony Landmarks

Arch: a deep projection, such as the vertebral arch.

Canal: a duct or channel, such as the ear canal.

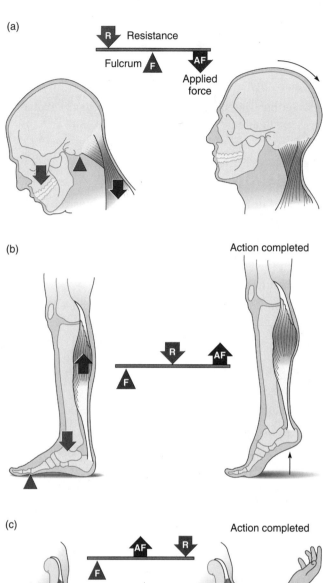

(a)

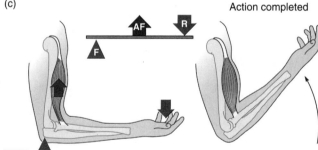

FIGURE 8.3
The lever system. **(a)** First-class lever. **(b)** Second-class lever. **(c)** Third-class lever. (Modified with permission from Premkumar K. The Massage Connection: Anatomy and Physiology, 2nd ed. Baltimore: Lippincott Williams & Wilkins; 2004. Fig. 4.11.)

Cartilage: firm, smooth, resilient nonvascular tissue.

Condyle: a rounded projection at the articulation of an extremity, such as the condyle of the humerus.

Crest: a bony ridge, such as the iliac crest.

Epicondyle: a bony projection on either side of a condyle area, such as the distal end of the humerus; it serves as an attachment point for muscles and ligaments.

Facet: a smooth plane surface, such as the articulation of the vertebrae.

Fissure: a cleft or groove, such as the anal fissure.

Foramen: an opening for nerves or other tissue to pass through, such as the vertebral foramen.

Fossa: a cavity or slight depression, such as the temporal fossa on the skull.

Greater trochanter: the large bony projection on the femur.

Groove: a furrow or channel, such as the laminar groove.

Head: the larger, thicker, heavier part of a bone, such as the head of the femur.

Line: a long, narrow ridge, such as the linea aspera of the femur.

Meatus: a natural passage or canal, such as the external auditory meatus.

Notch: a wide, shallow depression, such as the sternal notch.

Process: a projection, such as the coracoid process.

Sinus: a cavity within an organ or area, such as the nasal sinus.

Spinous process: a sharp, slender projection, such as the spine.

Sulcus: a groove along a bone that accommodates a nerve, tendon, or blood vessel, such as the intertubercular sulcus of the humerus.

Tubercle: a knob, such as that found on the posterior surface of a rib at the articulation of the transverse process.

Tuberosity: a rounded elevation, such as the ischial tuberosity.

The Bony Features of the Skull

Coronal suture: a line where the frontal section meets the two parietal sections of the skull.

Cranium: the general term for the eight bones of the head; together with the 14 bones of the face they make up the skull.

Ethmoid: the complex bone where the olfactory nerves pass through the cranium.

Fontanel: the junction in the skull where the coronal and sagittal sutures meet; it is membranous at birth.

Frontal bone: the forehead; the anterior part of the skull.

Inferior nasal concha: the thin curvy bones on the lateral sides of the nasal cavity.

Lacrimal: the bone where the glands that secrete tears are located.

Lambdoidal suture: the junction of the occipital and parietal bones.

Mandible: the lower jaw bone.

Mastoid: a bony process located at the lateral side of the skull, behind the ear.

Maxilla: the upper jaw bone.

Nasal: pertaining to the nose.

Occipital: referring to the back part of the head bones.

Ossicles: small bones of the ears.

Palatine: a pair of bones located in the back of the mouth.

Parietal: referring to the side bones of the skull.

Sagittal suture: the suture between the two parietal bones.

Sphenoid: a wedge-shaped bone in front of the occipital bone.

Squamous suture: the overlapping bone margins on the lateral side of the head.

Temporal: a large, irregular bone situated in the base and side of the skull.

Vomer: the partitioning bone between the nostrils.

Zygomatic: the bone beneath the orbit forming the cheek.

Bones of the Body

Atlas: the first vertebra; the head sits on it.

Axis: the second vertebra; allows side-to-side movement of the head.

Carpal: the wrist bone.

Clavicle: the collarbone.

Coccyx: the tailbone.

Femur: the thigh bone.

Fibula: the smaller, outer lower leg bone.

Humerus: the upper arm bone.

Metacarpals: the hand bones between the wrist and the fingers.

Metatarsals: the mid-bones of the foot, in between the ankle and the toes.

Patella: the kneecap.

Pelvic girdle: the hip bones.

Phalanges: the finger and toe bones.

Radius: the lower arm bone on the lateral aspect (thumb side) of the forearm.

Ribs: articulating from the spine, most of the bones that connect to the sternum to protect the thoracic organs.

Scapula: the shoulder blade.

Sternum: the breast bone.

Tibia: the larger, inner lower leg bone.

Ulna: the lower arm bone on the medial aspect (little finger side) of the forearm.

Vertebrae: the bones of the back (spinal column).

The Spine

The **spinal column** is the main support of the skeletal structure. It consists of vertebrae that are linked by intervertebral discs and held together by ligaments. There are seven **cervical** (neck) **vertebrae,** 12 **thoracic vertebrae,** and five **lumbar vertebrae** that are moveable. Five vertebrae are fused together to form the **sacrum,** and between three and five vertebrae are fused together to form the **coccyx** (Fig. 8.4). The vertebrae are made up of a bony body **(centrum)** that is cylindrical in shape, a transverse process on each side, a spinous process in the center, and an

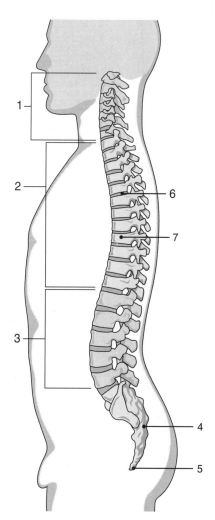

FIGURE 8.4
The spinal column from the side. *1:* Cervical vertebrae. *2:* Thoracic vertebrae. *3:* Lumbar vertebrae. *4:* Sacrum. *5:* Coccyx. *6:* Intervertebral disc. *7:* Vertebra. (Reprinted with permission from Cohen BJ, Wood DL. Memmler's The Human Body in Health and Disease, 9th ed. Philadelphia: Lippincott Williams & Wilkins; 2000. Fig. 19-3.)

arch. The arches enclose a cylindrical space called the **vertebral canal,** which houses the spinal cord and the spinal meninges, the covering around the cord. The 31 pairs of **spinal nerves** are formed by the union of the dorsal and ventral spinal nerve roots from each segment of the spinal cord. The **annulus fibrosus** is a ring of fibrous cartilage and tissue that forms the circumference of the intervertebral disc.

Curvatures of the Spine

Some pathological conditions are unique to the spine. Massage therapists often are confronted with clients who have abnormal curvatures of the spine. The following definitions are important:

Kyphosis: a posterior curvature of the thoracic spine, also called hunchback.

Lordoscoliosis: a combination of a posterior curvature of the lumbar area and a lateral curvature.

Lordosis: an anterior curvature of the lumbar area of the spine, also called swayback.

Scoliosis: a lateral curvature of the spine.

Another common affliction among massage therapy clients is a "slipped" or herniated disc, also referred to as a "bulging" disc, in the spinal column (Fig. 8.5). Although massage therapists are not allowed to diagnose, I find that when I am standing over the body of my prone clients, I often see obvious spinal misalignments. I refer a lot of clients to the chiropractor, who in turn refers clients to me.

Remember that except in cases of injury, disease, or birth defect, bones are often pulled out of alignment by shortened muscles. Massage is not about "tight muscles,"

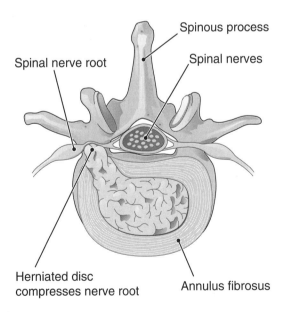

FIGURE 8.5

A herniated disc. (Reprinted with permission from Cohen BJ. Medical Terminology, 4th ed. Philadelphia: Lippincott, Williams & Wilkins; 2003. Fig. 19.13.)

it is about "shortened muscles," and the massage therapist's task is to lengthen them back to a neutral position. Even spinal curvatures often can be helped by lengthening the muscles inside the curvature. We can't claim to cure scoliosis, but we can help people who have it.

PATHOLOGY OF THE SKELETAL SYSTEM

The pathology of the skeletal system is an interesting and varied area of study. Because there are 206 bones in the body, all having their own functions, there is a lot of opportunity for injury and/or disease. More than 100 diseases fall under the general heading of **cancer,** three main types of which can affect the bones. **Osteosarcoma** is the most common type of bone cancer; it usually affects the extremities and most often occurs in children and adolescents. **Chondrosarcoma** develops in the cartilage, usually around the pelvis or extremities and usually affects middle-aged adults. **Ewing's sarcoma** begins in the immature cells of the bone marrow and usually affects children and adolescents. The pelvis, ribs, and extremities are the usual sites for cancer of this type.

Common bone conditions are the result of insult and/or trauma to the bone:

Dislocation: the displacement of a bone from its normal location.

Subluxation: a partial displacement of *one* of the bones that comprises a joint.

Compound fracture: a fracture in which the skin is broken and there is an open wound down to bone; sometimes referred to as an open fracture.

Closed fracture: a fracture in which the skin is intact at the break.

Other conditions may be **chronic** and not attributable to a particular injury, although they could be aggravated by an injury. Conversely, having one of these conditions could make a person more prone to injury because of lack of mobility:

Arthritis: an inflammation of the joints. The two most common forms are rheumatoid arthritis (an inflammatory destructive disease of the joints) and osteoarthritis (caused by the breakdown and eventual loss of the cartilage around the joints).

Gout: recurring episodes of arthritis in the peripheral joints, usually the big toe, caused by an excess of uric acid building up in the joint spaces.

Hyperparathyroidism: an endocrine disorder in which too much calcium is removed from the bone and put into the blood, which in turn causes bone pain; can also result in osteoporosis and pathologic fractures.

Osteoarthritis: Degeneration and eventual loss of the cartilage that serves as a cushion between the joints and bones; the resulting friction between bones causes pain and limits mobility. It occurs mainly in older people.

Osteomyelitis: an inflammation of the bone caused by a pus-producing organism; it may involve only a superficial area but is capable of penetrating through the bone.

Osteonecrosis: bone death resulting from poor blood supply to an area of bone.

Paget's disease: a disease in which the body loses bone marrow mass and replaces it with fibrous or vascular tissue.

Perth's disease: a deterioration of the head of the femur at the hip joint caused by a lack of blood supply; usually occurs during childhood and primarily affects boys.

Tips for Passing

Pay a lot of attention to this chapter, particularly the joints, the bony landmarks, and the pathology related to bones. This guide is not intended to be an anatomy book. Get your anatomy book out now and turn to the chapter on the skeletal system. Look at the pictures! You should be able to identify all the major bones of the body (by major, I mean anything longer than a few centimeters). If it's a bone, you need to know its name and its location. Stand in front of a full-length mirror and touch all the bones while naming them. Do the same thing with the muscles.

Affirmation

I have confidence in my own abilities.

Practice Questions

1. The human body has _____ bones.
   a. 198
   b. 226
   c. 196
   d. 206

2. Which of the following is an example of a long bone?
   a. Femur
   b. Greater trochanter
   c. Metatarsal
   d. Sternum

3. The hyoid is a(an)
   a. Long bone
   b. Irregularly shaped bone
   c. Cuboid
   d. Short bone

4. Which term refers to the joint where two bones meet?
   a. Cartilage
   b. Articulation
   c. Tuberosity
   d. Process

5. Immovable joints are classified as
   a. Synarthrotic
   b. Diarthrotic
   c. Amphiarthrotic
   d. Biarthrotic

6. An example of a freely movable joint is the
   a. Coronal suture
   b. Sacroiliac
   c. Hip
   d. Xiphoid

7. The _____ function(s) as a fulcrum.
   a. Joint
   b. Tendon
   c. Muscle
   d. Blood cells

8. The most plentiful levers in the body are
   a. First class
   b. Second class
   c. Third class
   d. Fourth class

9. A meatus is
   a. A thick muscle
   b. A crack in the bone
   c. A canal
   d. Part of the abdominal wall

10. The coronal and sagittal sutures meet at the
    a. Ethmoid
    b. Nasal concha
    c. Mastoid
    d. Fontanel

CHAPTER 9

The Muscular System

Long I thought that knowledge alone would suffice me—O if I could but obtain knowledge!

—Walt Whitman

HIGHLIGHTS

The study of the muscular system is known as **myology.** Muscles are often named according to their characteristics, such as their location, action, shape, position, relative size, and direction. The three types of muscle are skeletal, smooth, and cardiac. **Skeletal muscles,** also called *striated* (striped), are referred to as voluntary muscles because they enable conscious movements. **Smooth muscles** are nonstriated muscles that contract involuntarily; they line various internal organs and blood vessels. **Cardiac muscle** is found only in the heart and is striated, but also contracts involuntarily.

The function of the muscular system is movement. Without muscles, the skeleton would be frozen in space. Muscles convert the body's fuel into motion. They function in two ways: they **contract** (tighten) and **relax.** Muscles also stabilize body positions, regulate organ volume, move substances through the body, and produce heat for the body. The superficial muscles of the body are shown in Figure 9.1. Refer to your anatomy text for more detailed drawings.

The NCE includes questions pertaining to the insertion and origin of specific muscles (Table 9.1). The point where the muscle attaches to the stationary bone is normally referred to as the **origin.** The origin is usually closest to the trunk of the body, or proximal. The point where the muscle attaches to the moving bone is distal from the trunk and is referred to as the **insertion.** The mid-portion of the muscle, or fleshy part

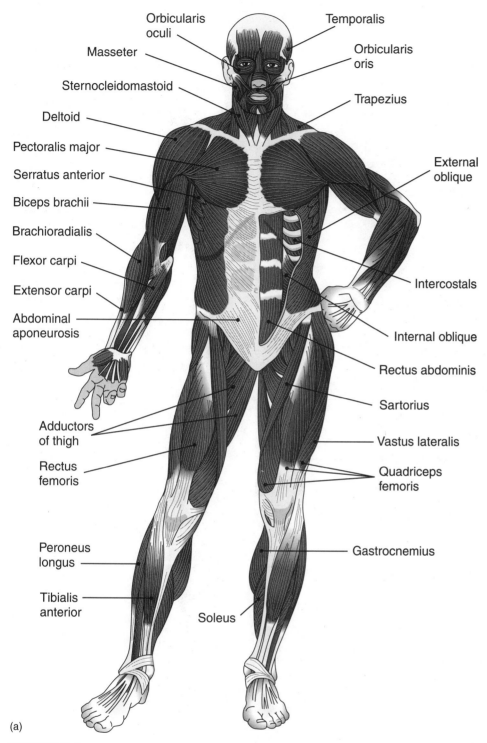

Orbicularis
oculi

Temporalis

Masseter

Orbicularis
oris

Sternocleidomastoid

Trapezius

Deltoid

Pectoralis major

External
oblique

Serratus anterior

Biceps brachii

Brachioradialis

Flexor carpi

Intercostals

Extensor carpi

Abdominal
aponeurosis

Internal oblique

Rectus abdominis

Sartorius

Adductors
of thigh

Vastus lateralis

Rectus
femoris

Quadriceps
femoris

Peroneus
longus

Gastrocnemius

Tibialis
anterior

Soleus

(a)

FIGURE 9.1
Superficial muscles. **(a)** Anterior view. *(continues)*

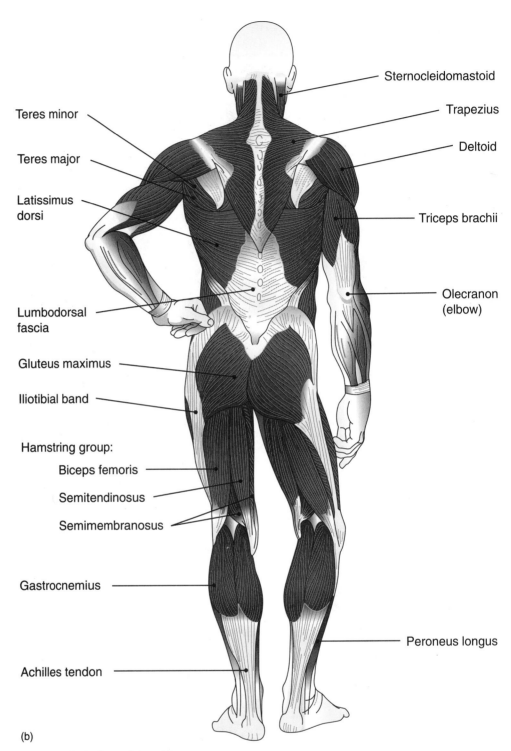

(b)

FIGURE 9.1 *(continued)*
(b) Posterior view. (Reprinted with permission from Cohen BJ, Wood DL. Memmler's The Human Body in Health and Disease, 9th ed. Philadelphia: Lippincott Williams & Wilkins; 2000. Figs. 20.3, 20.4.)

TABLE 9.1   The Origins and Insertions of Selected Muscles

Muscle	Origin	Insertion
Adductor longus and brevis	Anterior pubis	Linea aspera of posterior femur
Adductor magnus	Pubic ramus, ischial tuberosity	Linea aspera of posterior femur, adductor tubercle of medial femur
Anconeus	Lateral epicondyle of humerus	Olecranon process of ulna
Biceps brachii	Short head: coracoid process of scapula Long head: supraglenoid tubercle of scapula	Tuberosity of radius
Brachialis	Lower half of anterior shaft of humerus	Tuberosity of ulna
Brachioradialis	Lateral supracondylar ridge of humerus	Styloid process of radius
Buccinator	Maxilla, mandible	Lips
Deltoids	Anterior: lateral third of clavicle Middle: lateral acromion Posterior: spine of scapula	Deltoid tuberosity of humerus
Extensor digitorum longus	Lateral epicondyle of tibia, proximal two-thirds of anterior shaft of fibula	Middle and distal phalanges of 4 lateral toes
External oblique	Lower 8 ribs	Abdominal aponeurosis and iliac crest
Gastrocnemius	Medial head: medial epicondyle of femur Lateral head: lateral epicondyle of femur	Calcaneus via Achilles tendon
Gluteus maximus	Posterior sacrum, ilium, superior gluteal line of ilium	Gluteal tuberosity of femur and iliotibial tract
Gluteus medius	Iliac crest, ilium between superior and middle gluteal lines	Greater trochanter
Gracilis	Anterior pubis	Medial proximal tibia
Hamstrings	Biceps femoris, long head: ischial tuberosity; short head: linea aspera Semitendinosus and semimembranosis: ischial tuberosity	Biceps femoris: head of fibula Semitendinosus: posterior medial tibial condyle Semimembranosus: anterior proximal tibial shaft
Iliacus	Inner surface of ilium	Lesser trochanter
Infraspinatus	Infraspinous fossa of scapula	Greater tubercle of humerus
Internal oblique	Inguinal ligament and anterior iliac crest	Costal cartilages of last 4 ribs, abdominal aponeurosis
Latissimus dorsi	Thoracic lumbar aponeurosis from T7 to iliac crest, spinous processes Lower 3–4 ribs Inferior angle of scapula	Bicipital groove of humerus
Levator scapula	C1–C4 transverse processes	Vertebral border of scapula from superior angle to root of spine
Masseter	Zygomatic arch	Mandible

continued

TABLE 9.1 The Origins and Insertions of Selected Muscles *(Continued)*

Muscle	Origin	Insertion
Orbicularis oris	Maxilla, mandible, lips, buccinator	Mucuous membranes, muscles inserting into lips
Pectoralis major	Clavicular head at medial half of clavicle Sternal head at sternum Cartilage of upper 6 ribs	Lateral lip of bicipital groove of the humerus
Pectoralis minor	Anterior 3–5 ribs	Coracoid process of scapula
Peroneus longus	Lateral shaft of fibula	Base of first metatarsal and first (medial) cuneiform, plantar surface
Psoas major	T12 and lumbar vertebrae	Lesser trochanter
Rectus abdominis	Costal cartilages 5, 6, 7	Pubis
Rhomboid major	T2–T5 spinous processes	Vertebral border at the root of the spine of the scapula
Rhomboid minor	C7 and T1, spinous processes	Root of spine of scapula
Sartorius	Anterior superior iliac spine (ASIS)	Upper medial shaft of tibia
Serratus anterior	Outer surface of upper 8 ribs	Vertebral border of scapula
Soleus	Soleal line of tibia, posterior head, and upper shaft of fibula	Calcaneus via Achilles tendon
Sternocleidomastoid	Manubrium of sternum	Mastoid process and clavicle
Subclavius	First rib	Inferior shaft of clavicle
Subscapularis	Subscapular fossa of scapula	Lesser tubercle of humerus
Supraspinatus	Supraspinous fossa of scapula	Greater tubercle of humerus
Temporalis	Lateral surface of temporal bone	Mandible
Tensor fascia latae	Iliac crest	Iliotibial tract
Teres major	Inferior angle of scapula	Medial tip of bicipital groove of humerus
Teres minor	Upper axillary border of scapula	Greater tubercle of humerus
Tibialis anterior	Lateral shaft of tibia, interosseous membrane	Base of first metatarsal, first cuneiform
Trapezius	Occiput, ligamentem nuchae, C1–T12	Upper-lateral clavicle, acromion Middle-spine of scapula Lower-root of spine of scapula
Triceps brachii	Long head: infraglenoid tubercle of scapula Short head: posterior humerus above spiral groove Medial head: posterior humerus below spinal groove	Olecranon process of ulna

between the insertion and origin, is normally referred to as the **belly,** as shown in Figure 9.2.

There are 630 active muscles in the body, and they work in groups to produce movement. From the perspective of a massage therapist working with a client who is in pain or whose body is out of balance, remember this: *muscles never push on other muscles; they are only pulled upon by shortened muscles.* Keep in mind that massage therapy is not about tight muscles; it is about lengthening shortened muscles and restoring the muscle to its proper place.

In addition to origins and insertions, the NCE contains questions about function and the potential relationship between muscles and pathology. To understand how the muscles function, you should focus on the relationship between the agonist, the antagonist, and the synergist. The **agonist,** also known as the prime mover, is the main muscle that contracts to perform an action. The **antagonist** is the opposing muscle that stretches and yields to the actions of the agonist. The **synergist(s)** is a muscle that contracts to stabilize intermediate joints either to help prevent unwanted movements or to aid the movement of the agonist.

Muscle is surrounded by **fascia,** or connective tissue. Fascia occurs in multiple layers and serves multiple purposes. The **superficial fascia** keeps the muscles separated from the skin. **Adipose fascia** holds in body temperature and serves as muscle protection. **Deep fascia** lines the body walls and holds related muscles together in addition to carrying blood and lymph vessels. Rising from the fascia are three more layers. The outer layer, the **epimysium,** covers the whole muscle. The center layer, the **perimysium,** surrounds muscle fibers that are separated into groups called **fascicles** of anywhere from 10 to more than 100. The third, thin sheet of connective tissue, the **endomysium,** surrounds the inside of each fascicle and separates the individual muscle fibers, which are composed of **myofibrils,** from each other (Fig. 9.3). These tissue layers mesh at the **musculotendinous junctions** with the connective tissue that forms **tendons,** the cords of thick tissue that serve as the attachments between skeletal muscle and bone. If the connective tissue stretches over a broad, flat area, such as on the heel or the top of the head, it is referred to as an **aponeurosis.**

Muscle tissue has four specific characteristics that enable it to function. **Electrical excitability** is the ability to respond to stimuli by producing electrical signals. **Contractility** is the muscle's ability to contract when stimulated by a nerve signal. **Extensibility** is the ability of the muscle to stretch without being damaged. **Elasticity** is the ability of the muscle to return to its original shape and length after is has been contracted or extended.

Muscles are composed of multiple **fibers.** The number of muscles in a developing embryo is the same number of muscles an adult will have. The growth that occurs in muscles after birth is just an enlargement of existing fibers. Muscles are made up of three different kinds of proteins. **Myosin** and **actin** are **contractile proteins,** which produce force during muscle contractions. **Regulatory proteins,** such as **tropomyosin** and **troponin,** act by switching muscle contractions on and off. **Structural proteins** aid in elasticity and extensibility.

The **motor unit** controls muscle contraction and is composed of a **motor neuron** plus all the skeletal muscle fibers it can stimulate. A **twitch** occurs when all the muscle fibers in a motor unit contract in response to a single nerve signal in the motor neuron. Twitches can also be produced by electrical stimulation.

Nerve signals are transmitted across the gap, or **synapse,** between a motor neuron and a muscle fiber; in skeletal muscle, the synapse is known as the **neuromuscular**

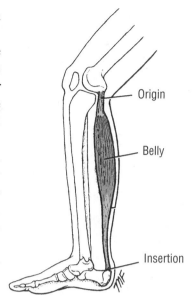

Origin

Belly

Insertion

FIGURE 9.2
Origin, insertion, and belly of the gastrocnemius muscle. (Modified with permission from Snell RS. Clinical Anatomy. 7th ed. Baltimore: Lippincott Williams & Wilkins; 2003. Fig. 1.9.)

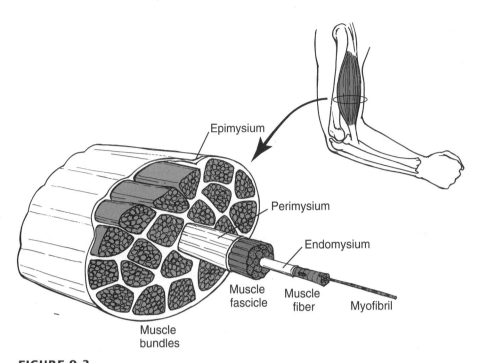

FIGURE 9.3
Anatomy of a muscle showing the layers of the connective tissue. (Reprinted with permission from Hendrickson T. Massage for Orthopedic Conditions. Baltimore: Lippincott Williams & Wilkins; 2003. Fig. 1.15.)

junction. There are two primary types of muscle fibers: slow-twitch and fast-twitch. Some muscle fibers are referred to as **slow-twitch fibers** because they are tiny and contract slowly. Slow-twitch fibers are capable of prolonged contraction—for instance, enabling us to stand for hours. **Fast-twitch fibers** are much larger in diameter and can produce the most powerful muscle contractions, but they fatigue quickly. Fast-twitch fibers facilitate short bursts of activity, such as the movements of aerobic exercise. During exercise, the body takes in extra oxygen to sustain prolonged periods of muscle contraction. Immediately after exercise, deep breathing maintains oxygen at a higher level than is necessary during rest. The extra oxygen is needed to pay off the **oxygen debt** incurred while performing strenuous activity.

In skeletal muscle, **muscle tone** is caused by an alternating pattern of motor units being active and inactive, resulting in keeping the muscle firm without causing any action. Muscle fibers also have a characteristic known as the **all-or-none response**. This means that a stimulus must be strong enough to excite the entire fiber—or none of the muscle fiber will react. When thinking of muscle movements, it is helpful to remember certain terminology (Fig. 9.4). **Adduction** "adds" to the body—in other words, the bone (and therefore, muscle) is coming closer to the midline. **Abduction** makes the bone "absent," or away from the midline. **Flexion** decreases the angle of a joint. When flexing the biceps, you are making a 45-degree angle from an angle that was 90 degrees, assuming the arm was fully **extended.** A **levator** acts like an **elevator,** raising something up, and a **depressor** does just the opposite. A **tensor** generates force to allow the muscle to perform certain actions. **Inversion** turns inward; **eversion** turns outward. **Supination** turns upward (supine); **pronation** turns downward (prone).

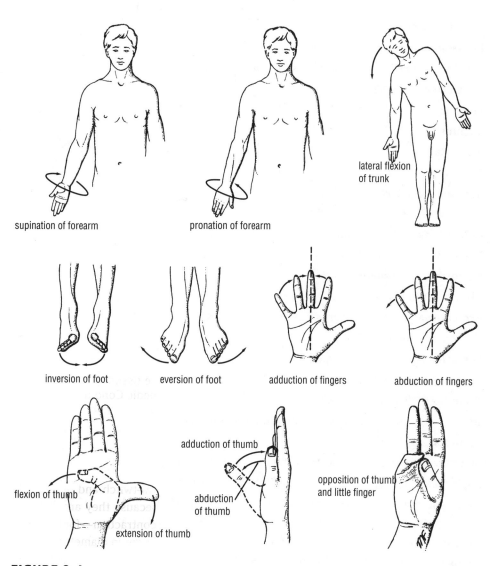

FIGURE 9.4
Terminology used in relation to movement. (Reprinted with permission from Snell RS. Clinical Anatomy. 7th ed. Baltimore: Lippincott Williams & Wilkins; 2003. Fig. 1.3.)

WHAT YOU NEED TO KNOW

Abductor: a muscle that moves bone away from the midline.

Adductor: a muscle that moves bone closer to the midline.

Agonist: the main muscle that contracts to perform an action; also known as the prime mover.

Antagonist: the opposing muscle that stretches and yields to the actions of the agonist.

Biceps: having two heads.

Brevis: shortest.

Deltoid: triangular in shape.

Depressor: a muscle that produces inferior motions.

Extensor: a muscle that increases the angle of a joint.

Flexor: a muscle that decreases the angle of a joint.

Gracilis: slender.

Latissimus: widest.

Levator: a muscle that produces superior motions.

Longissimus: longest.

Longus: long.

Magnus: large.

Major: larger.

Maximus: largest.

Minimus: smallest.

Oblique: diagonal to the midline.

Orbicularis: circular in shape.

Pectinate: comb-like.

Piriformis: pear-shaped.

Platys: flat in shape.

Pronator: a muscle that turns inferiorly or posteriorly.

Quadratus: square in shape.

Quadriceps: having four heads.

Rectus: parallel to the midline.

Rhomboid: diamond-shaped.

Rotator: a muscle that moves bone around a longitudinal axis.

Serratus: saw-toothed.

Sphincter: a muscle that decreases the size of an opening.

Supinator: a muscle that turns superiorly or anteriorly.

Synergist: a muscle that contracts to stabilize intermediate joints to either help prevent unwanted movements or aid the movement of the agonist.

Tensor: a muscle that holds a body part rigid.

Transverse: perpendicular to the midline.

Trapezius: trapezoid in shape.

Triceps: having three heads.

PATHOLOGY OF THE MUSCULAR SYSTEM

Generally speaking, there are only a few causes of pathological changes in the muscles: trauma caused by injury; ischemia (lack of oxygen to the muscle); and nerve or genetic problems, which may include diseases, myopathies, dystrophies, and other disorders. As when working with any serious condition, it is wise to check with the client's doctor if there is any concern that bodywork may be contraindicated. When working with a client who has sustained an injury, the massage therapist must get a doctor's release before proceeding with the bodywork if bones have been broken and/or soft tissue has been compromised. For injuries such as **strains** or **sprains,** give the body time to rest and heal before performing bodywork, usually at least 48 hours. This is the **acute** phase. **RICE (rest, ice, compression, elevation)** is probably necessary for a day or two before the client has massage or bodywork. If there is any doubt that massage might cause further injury, check with the physician before proceeding.

A **sprain** is a stretching or tearing of a ligament; it may simply be overextended or may be fully torn, in which case surgery will be required to mend it. A **strain** is a tearing of the muscle itself and is usually less serious than a sprain. Strains and sprains are classified as first, second, or third degree. A first-degree strain or sprain is not serious; the fibers have only been stretched and not torn. Pain, swelling, and limitations will be minimal. A second-degree sprain or strain is more serious, involving a partial tear and accompanied by moderate pain, swelling, and some limitation. A third-degree sprain or strain is the most serious, involving a complete tear of the tissue, severe pain and swelling, and a marked degree of limitation.

Myopathy is a general term that refers to any disease in the muscle. **Muscular atrophy,** which can result from injury or disease, is a progressive weakening of the muscle caused by degenerating neurons. Although massage therapy may not reverse atrophy, it is still beneficial because of the mechanical effect of the increase in circulation. One therapist I know reports that her most satisfying experience is working on a quadriplegic young man. Although he cannot "feel" the bodywork, he looks forward to it immensely and is well aware of the benefits he receives through the sessions. It is like exercise for people who can't do it themselves. Clients with **chronic conditions** (lasting 3 months or longer) such as fibromyalgia, multiple sclerosis, rheumatoid arthritis, or osteoarthritis can greatly benefit from receiving regular massage.

Muscular dystrophy is a collective term for diseases that cause a progressive loss of muscle fibers without any nervous system involvement. Most dystrophies are caused by a gene mutation that affects the body's ability to metabolize certain nutrients. **Duchenne muscular dystrophy (DMD),** the most common form, causes muscles to tear easily and to slowly rupture and die. DMD affects only males, and life expectancy is age 20 to 30 for those who have it.

A **myoma** is a benign tumor composed of muscle tissue. **Myositis** refers to inflammation of muscle. In **myositis ossificans,** muscle tissue accumulates calcium deposits and begins to harden. A **contracture** is a permanent shortening of a muscle. **Volkmann's contracture** is a permanent shortening of a muscle caused by damaged or destroyed muscle fibers being replaced by scar tissue, usually caused by a lack of circulation from some outside interference such as a cast or elastic bandage that is too tight. **Dupuytren's contracture** is a painless thickening of the fascia in the palm of the hand that results in the inability to move the digits. Dupuytren's may be genetic or may be caused by injury.

Trigger points, sometimes incorrectly referred to as tender points or trigger zones, are tender areas of hyperirritability that cause sensations to be referred to an area outside of the specific tenderness, referred to as a spillover zone (Fig. 9.5). Many conditions aggravate trigger points. People who have **fibromyalgia** (literally, pain in the fibers) and other chronic conditions often have many active trigger points. Trigger points frequently accompany stress and tension held in the body.

Other pathological conditions of the muscles with which you should be familiar are listed here.

Acquired metabolic and toxic myopathies: damage to muscle caused by environmental toxins or by a failure of the body to metabolize certain nutrients; not a genetic condition.

Anterior compartment syndrome: another term for mild shin splints, a tendinitis of the anterior compartment muscles of the leg that flex the foot; also can be more serious than shin splints.

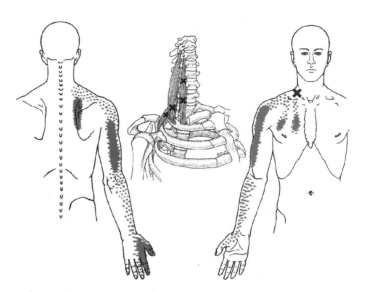

FIGURE 9.5
Trigger points of the anterior, medius, and posterior right scalene are indicated by *Xs. Solid shading* indicates the essential referred pain zones. *Stippling* maps the spillover zones. (Reprinted with permission from MediClip image, copyright © 2003. Baltimore: Lippincott Williams & Wilkins.)

Chronic fatigue syndrome: a chronic condition characterized by severe chronic fatigue of 6 months or longer duration; linked to the Epstein–Barr virus.

Cramp/spasm: an unusually painful muscle contraction.

Flaccidity: muscles that are weak, lax, or soft.

Hernia: a protrusion of an organ or other tissue through an abnormal opening in the wall of the cavity normally containing it, or in soft tissue.

Plantar fasciitis: inflammation of the plantar fascia on the sole of the foot; very painful.

Poliomyelitis: an acute viral disease that may end in permanent muscle atrophy and contracture.

Post-polio syndrome: a neuromuscular syndrome that may develop years after recovery from polio.

Rotator cuff tear: a tear in one of the rotator cuff muscles (teres minor, subscapularis, supraspinatus, infraspinatus); makes abduction and rotation painful.

Shin splint: tenderness, swelling, and pain of the anterior leg muscles; a mild form of anterior compartment syndrome.

Spasticity: a condition characterized by increased muscle tone in which abnormal stretch reflexes intensify muscle resistance to passive movements.

Tendinitis: inflammation of tendons and muscle attachments.

Tenosynovitis: inflammation of the tendon sheath (covering).

Torticollis: a contracted state of the cervical muscles, producing a twisted neck and unnatural head position; sometimes referred to as "wry neck."

Tips for Passing

Try this when studying with a partner. At the massage school I attended, the students would draw the muscles onto each other using grease pencils. It is a great hands-on way to learn. Rub massage cream onto the body first and the grease will wash right off when you're finished.

Practice Questions

1. The point where muscle attaches to the moving bone is referred to as the
   a. Belly
   b. Origin
   c. Insertion
   d. Fascia

2. The connective tissue that binds muscles together is the
   a. Membrane
   b. Fascitis
   c. Fascia
   d. Dermatome

3. Lack of oxygen to the muscle causes
   a. Ischemia
   b. Myositis
   c. Cyanide poisoning
   d. Halitosis

4. RICE is the acronym for
   a. Redness, ischemia, compression, elevation
   b. Rest, ice, compression, elevation
   c. Redness, ice, compression, exercise
   d. Rest, ice, compression, exercise

5. The fleshy part of a muscle is the
   a. Origin
   b. Insertion
   c. Belly
   d. End plate

6. A progressive loss of muscle fibers without any nervous system involvement is caused by
   a. Multiple sclerosis
   b. Muscular dystrophy
   c. Huntington's disease
   d. Cerebral palsy

7. A progressive weakening of the muscle caused by degenerating neurons is
   a. Muscular atrophy
   b. Muscular contractions
   c. Ferrous muscularity
   d. Ischemia

8. The study of the muscular system is called
   a. Skeletology
   b. Anatomy

Affirmation

As I remember to breathe deeply and slowly, I am exhaling any stress on the test with every breath. I feel the stress leaving my body.

    c. Myology

    d. Osteopathy

9. The condition in which the tendon sheath is inflamed is called

    a. Shin splints

    b. Sprain

    c. Tendonitis

    d. Tenosynovitis

10. The number of muscles in the human body is

    a. 1002

    b. 630

    c. 206

    d. 302

CHAPTER 10

The Nervous System

Many a poor sore-eyed student that I have heard of would grow faster,
both intellectually and physically, if, instead of sitting up so very late, he
honestly slumbered a fool's allowance.

—HENRY DAVID THOREAU

HIGHLIGHTS

The structure of the nervous system actually encompasses two different but interrelated systems: the central nervous system and the peripheral nervous system. The **central nervous system (CNS)** includes the **brain** and the **spinal cord** and is the control center of the body. The **peripheral nervous system (PNS)** refers to all outlying nervous tissue, such as the **cranial nerves, spinal nerves,** and **sensory receptors.** The PNS is divided into nerve **plexuses,** or networks of intersecting nerves (Table 10.1). **Dermatomes** are areas of skin innervated by a single spinal nerve, as shown in Figure 10.1.

In humans and many other animals, the function of the nervous system is to work in close relationship with the endocrine system, responding to sensory input and adjusting accordingly. The PNS is subdivided into the **somatic nervous system,** which controls skeletal muscle contractions; the **autonomic nervous system (ANS)**, which regulates smooth muscles, cardiac muscle, the internal organs, and glands; and the enteric nervous system. The **enteric nervous system,** referred to as "the brain of the gut," controls the gastrointestinal (GI) tract, including its muscle contractions and secretions. The ANS has two divisions: the sympathetic nervous system and the parasympathetic nervous system. The **sympathetic nervous system** prepares the body for stress ("fight or flight") and the **parasympathetic nervous system** prepares the body for rest ("rest and digest").

Nervous tissue is composed of two main types of cells, neurons, and glia. **Neurons,**

TABLE 10.1   Plexuses of the Peripheral Nervous System

Cervical Plexus	Brachial Plexus	Lumbar Plexus	Sacral Plexus
Ansa cervicalis	Axillary	Femoral	Gluteal
Greater auricular	Dorsoscapular	Genitofemoral	Posterior femoral cutaneous
Lesser occipital	Long thoracic	Iliohypogastric	
Phrenic	Median	Ilioinguinal	Pudendal
Supraclavicular	Musculocutaneous	Lateral femoral cutaneous	Sciatic
Transverse cervical	Pectorals		
	Radial	Obturator	
	Subclavius		
	Subscapular		
	Suprascapular		
	Thoracodorsal		
	Ulnar		

or nerve cells, are the functional unit of the nervous system. Neurons are specialized cells that transmit electrical impulses from one part of the body to another. A neuron has two main components, dendrites, and glial cells. The **dendrite** receives incoming nerve impulses, and the **axon** carries nerve signals away from the body of the neuron. **Glial cells,** also known as neuroglia or glia, are supporting cells that provide electrical insulation, as well as other support functions.

Think of a group of neurons, or nerve fibers, as a telephone line. Messages in the neurons are carried along with the help of chemicals called **neurotransmitters.** The neurotransmitters are released from the tip of the axon into the **synapse** at the **synaptic cleft,** and they will either stimulate or inhibit the next neuron. **Acetylcholine** is a neurotransmitter that propagates electrical impulses from one nerve cell to another in the PNS. Acetylcholine is excitable at neuromuscular junctions in skeletal muscle but is inhibitory elsewhere, as in slowing down the heart rate. **Serotonin,** another neurotransmitter, is involved in the regulation of sleep, body temperature, and sensory perception but is also thought to have something to do with our moods. **Epinephrine, norepinephrine,** and **dopamine** are all in the same class as serotonin, called **biogenic amines.** Epinephrine and norepinephrine are hormones as well as neurotransmitters. All of them help regulate mood, as well as some of our biological functions.

Some neurotransmitters are composed of a single **amino acid,** but others are composed of as many as 40 amino acids that have bonded together. These are called **neuropeptides. Enkephalins** and **endorphins** are examples of neuropeptides. Both of these are vital to the body's physiology in many areas, but their primary function is as the body's natural painkillers. **Substance P** is a neurotransmitter that sends sensations of pain to the CNS, and enkephalins suppress them. The most common inhibitory neurotransmitter in the body is **GABA (gamma-aminobutyric acid).** GABA is present only in the brain, and approximately 30% of all brain synapses rely on GABA.

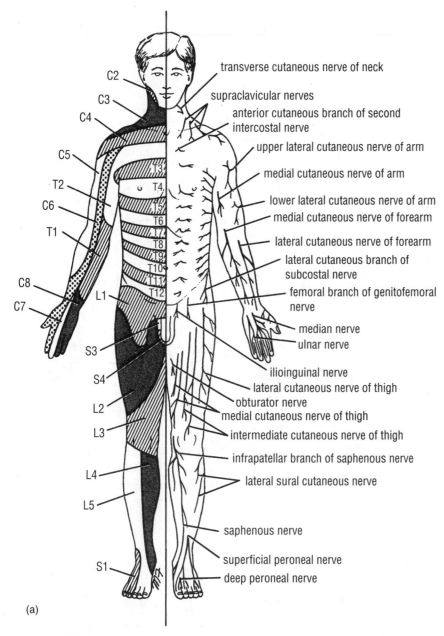

C2
C3
C4
C5
T2
C6
T1
C8
C7
S3
S4
L2
L3
L4
L5
S1

T3
T4
T5
T6
T7
T8
T9
T10
T11
T12
L1

transverse cutaneous nerve of neck

supraclavicular nerves

anterior cutaneous branch of second
intercostal nerve

upper lateral cutaneous nerve of arm

medial cutaneous nerve of arm

lower lateral cutaneous nerve of arm
medial cutaneous nerve of forearm

lateral cutaneous nerve of forearm

lateral cutaneous branch of
subcostal nerve

femoral branch of genitofemoral
nerve

median nerve
ulnar nerve

ilioinguinal nerve
lateral cutaneous nerve of thigh
obturator nerve
medial cutaneous nerve of thigh

intermediate cutaneous nerve of thigh

infrapatellar branch of saphenous nerve

lateral sural cutaneous nerve

saphenous nerve

superficial peroneal nerve
deep peroneal nerve

(a)

FIGURE 10.1
Dermatomes [on *left* in (a), on *right* in (b)] and the distribution of
cutaneous nerves [on *right* in (a), on *left* in (b)] on the body.

There are actually three different types of neurons, each one serving a different purpose. **Sensory neurons,** also called **afferent neurons,** usually have a long dendrite and a short axon, and carry messages from sensory receptors to the CNS. **Motor neurons,** also called **efferent neurons,** have short dendrites and long axons, and carry messages from the CNS to the muscles or glands. **Interneurons** transmit messages only between neurons.

Sensory neurons act on signals from the five senses: touch, taste, smell, sight, and hearing. **Chemoreceptors** are specialized cells that react to chemical substances and relay information throughout the CNS. They respond to outside stimuli, such as tastes

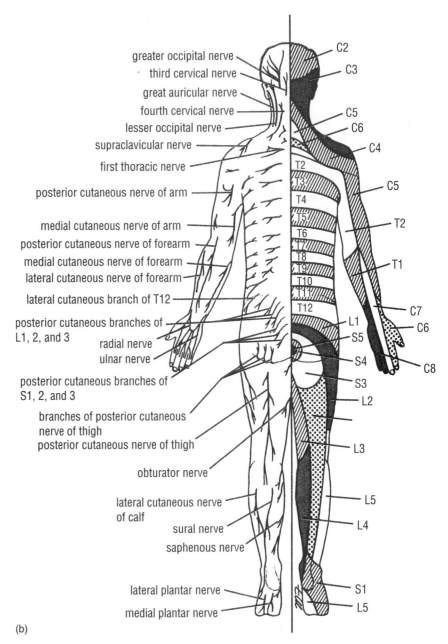

greater occipital nerve
third cervical nerve
great auricular nerve
fourth cervical nerve
lesser occipital nerve
supraclavicular nerve
first thoracic nerve
posterior cutaneous nerve of arm

medial cutaneous nerve of arm
posterior cutaneous nerve of forearm
medial cutaneous nerve of forearm
lateral cutaneous nerve of forearm
lateral cutaneous branch of T12
posterior cutaneous branches of
L1, 2, and 3
radial nerve
ulnar nerve
posterior cutaneous branches of
S1, 2, and 3
branches of posterior cutaneous
nerve of thigh
posterior cutaneous nerve of thigh

obturator nerve

lateral cutaneous nerve
of calf
sural nerve
saphenous nerve

lateral plantar nerve
medial plantar nerve

C2
C3

C5
C6
C4

C5
T2
T1

C7
C6
C8

L1
S5
S4
S3
L2

L3

L5
L4

S1
L5

(b)

FIGURE 10.1 *continued*

(a) Anterior view. (b) Posterior view. (Reprinted with permission from Snell
RS.Clinical Anatomy, 7th ed. Baltimore: Lippincott Williams & Wilkins; 2003.)

or smells, and internal stimuli, like the mixture of gases in the blood. **Photoreceptors**
respond to light on the retina of the eye. **Nociceptors** are free nerve endings that
respond to pain. **Thermoceptors** detect heat or cold. **Proprioceptors** are located
throughout the muscular and skeletal systems and provide information about body
movements and position. **Joint kinesthetic receptors** act the same as proprioceptors,
except they are exclusively located in the joints.

The nervous system is primarily a system of stimulus and response. There is a
reflex, or reflective action, for every stimulus. Reflexes are preprogrammed in the body
and do not require any conscious effort, although they can be overcome through

conscious effort. The **reflex arc** is the route through the nervous system that connects a receptor and an effector. Examples of the flexor reflex and the stretch reflex are shown in Figure 10.2. There are many different types of reflexes in the body (Table 10.2).

The study of the nervous system and its diseases and disorders is known as **neurology.** The nervous system is very complex and interrelated with other systems. The definitions address the nervous system in general. The brain and spinal cord are addressed more thoroughly in Chapter 11.

WHAT YOU NEED TO KNOW

Acetylcholine: a chemical that carries messages across the synaptic cleft at the synapse, the space between two neurons.

Action potential: the electrical signal that rapidly propagates along the axon of nerve cells and over the surface of some muscle and glandular cells. Action potentials sweep like a wave along axons to transfer information from one place to another in the nervous system.

All-or-none principle: the principle stating that muscle fibers always contract completely each time they are stimulated by their motor neuron, and that they do not contract at all if they are not stimulated by their motor neuron.

ATP (adenosine triphosphate): the universal energy storage molecule used as a ready energy source in all living cells for all biological energy needs.

Axolemma: the external plasma membrane of an axon.

Axon: the part of a neuron that carries messages away from the cell body toward target cells.

Axon hillock: the swelling of an axon where it joins a neuron's cell body; the place where action potentials (nerve impulses) are generated.

Axoplasm: the cytoplasm of a neuron.

Bipolar neuron: a neuron that has two projections arising from opposite ends of the cell body.

Chemical synapse: a gap between two neurons in the brain across which an

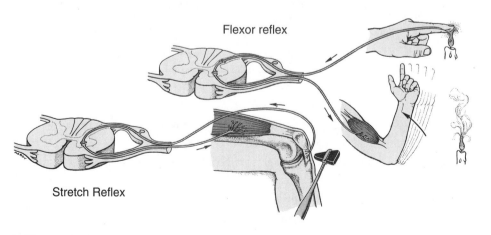

FIGURE 10.2

Reflex arcs. **Top:** A flexor reflex. **Bottom:** A stretch reflex. (Reprinted with permission of Neil O. Hardy, Westpoint, CT.)

TABLE 10.2	Reflexes
Reflex	**Definition**
Crossed reflex	Elicits a response on one side of the body when the opposite side is stimulated
Extensor thrust reflex	Extends the limbs whenever there is pressure applied to the surface of the hands or the feet
Flexor withdrawal reflex (also called nociceptive reflex)	Causes flexion of the lower extremity whenever the foot is painfully stimulated
Intersegmental reflex	A single sensory neuron activates more than one motor neuron, stimulating more than one effector, and causing more than one action to take place
Monosynaptic reflex	A direct neural connection between the sensory cells and the motor neuron with no intermediary neuron needed
Optical righting reflex	Allows humans (and other animals) to maintain the head in the correct position using the neck and limbs based on visual clues from the environment
Pilomotor reflex	Technical name for "goosebumps," a contraction of the smooth muscle of the skin because of cold or a very light stimulating touch
Postural reflex (also called righting reflex)	Works through the trunk and the extremities to keep the body at its right place in space when force is working to make it otherwise (such as falling)
Psychogalvanic reflex	A change in the electrical resistance of the skin caused by an emotional condition
Startle reflex	Contraction of the limb and neck muscles that occurs in response to being startled
Stretch reflex	Tonic contraction of the muscles due to an applied force; keeps a muscle from stretching far enough to be torn
Tendon reflex	Takes place deep in the muscle whenever tapotement (percussion) is applied to the attached tendon
Vasomotor reflex	Regulates the diameter of the blood vessels in response to varying degrees of sympathetic stimulation
Visceromotor reflex	Contraction of the muscles of the abdomen or thorax in response to a stimulus from an internal organ

impulse is transmitted by diffusion from one neuron to another neuron by means of a chemical neurotransmitter.

Chromatolysis: disintegration or damage to a part of a cell due to overexhaustion or injury.

Conduction: the transmission of nerve impulses or electricity.

Current: the amount of charge carried during a unit of time (minuscule, in the nervous system).

Dendrite: the receptive surface of a neuron; a thread-like projection like the branch of a tree.

Depolarization: movement of the membrane potential in the positive direction, from its normal negative level.

Dopamine: a chemical neurotransmitter *and* a hormone.

Electrical synapse: a junction where two excitable cells (neurons or muscle cells) meet.

Endorphin: a natural opiate produced by the brain to diminish pain.

Excitatory: causing an action to take place.

Excitotoxicity: the destruction of neurons caused by prolonged excitation of synaptic transmissions.

Glial cells: specialized cells that surround neurons, providing mechanical and physical support and electrical insulation; also called glia or neuroglia.

Grey matter: areas of the brain where thought takes place, composed mostly of nerve cell bodies and blood vessels.

Inhibitory: interrupting or preventing an action or secretion.

Membrane potential: the electrical potential difference across a membrane.

Multipolar neuron: a neuron that has numerous processes, usually an axon and three or more dendrites.

Myelin sheath: a layer of insulation that surrounds nerve fibers and speeds up the conduction of electrical impulses.

Norepinephrine: a hormone and also the neurotransmitter for most of the sympathetic nervous system.

Nucleus: the major organelle of a neuron.

Purkinje cell: an output neuron; Purkinje cells are the only ones that send signals away from the cerebellum.

Pyramidal cells: a type of neuron in the cerebral cortex that is shaped like a pyramid.

Refractory period: a "resting period" between nerve impulses; the time after a neuron fires or a muscle fiber contracts, during which a stimulus will not evoke a response.

Renshaw cell: an inhibitory interneuron.

Threshold: the point at which a stimulus first produces a response.

Unipolar neuron: a neuron with a single process (an axon, no dendrites) resulting from the fusion of two polar processes.

Unmyelinated: having no insulating sheath; unmyelinated neurons conduct impulses slowly.

White matter: the portion of the CNS, including the inner part of the cerebrum, which is made of nerve fibers, many of which are myelinated. The nerve fibers carry information as the nerve impulse between the brain and the spinal cord.

PATHOLOGY OF THE NERVOUS SYSTEM

The nervous system is highly complex, and a vast amount of pathology is associated with it—from congenital deformities to insult and injury. The pathology of the nervous system is known as **neuropathology.** The pathology of the CNS is different from that of the PNS, and still more pathological conditions will be covered in Chapter 11 on the brain and spinal cord. Here is a list of the most well-known neurological conditions associated with the CNS:

Alzheimer's disease: a progressive death of nerve cells, resulting in loss of function and memory; the cause is unknown.

Aneurysm: a pulsating, blood-filled sac protruding from the wall of a blood vessel or the heart.

Anxiety state: Anxiety is a feeling of unease and fear that can be characterized as endogenous (originating within) or exogenous (caused by some external factor). An anxiety state is usually characterized by hyperventilation, palpitations, sweating, and feelings of stress, and is usually temporary. Anxiety occurs in degrees; anxiety of a high magnitude may lead to a chronic panic disorder.

Blood clot: blood turned from a liquid to a solid by coagulation.

Central nervous system trauma: any injury causing malfunction of the CNS.

Cerebral palsy: a collection of motor disorders resulting from damage to the brain that occurred before, during, or after birth, causing impaired movements and slurred speech; not progressive but incurable.

Cerebrovascular accident (CVA): an impeded blood supply to some part of the brain, resulting in injury to brain tissue.

Chorea: a progressive loss of neuron function resulting in jerky, uncontrollable movements.

Cluster headache: a recurring headache that attacks several times a day for a period of days, followed by long periods during which the person is headache-free. There are two forms of cluster headache, episodic and chronic.

Complete transection: a severing of the spinal cord, resulting in loss of sensation and movement in all areas below the transection.

Concussion: a head injury severe enough to cause a loss of consciousness, seizure, amnesia, or changes in thought processes.

Contusion: an injury severe enough to cause a bruise without breaking the skin.

Degenerative disorder: any disorder in which the loss of ability or activity is progressive.

Dementia: a general loss of intellectual abilities and profound changes in personality; most often caused by Alzheimer's disease or other brain conditions, such as stroke or Parkinson's disease.

Depression: an emotional state characterized by sadness and despair; also used in medical contexts to indicate a loss of function (clinical depression).

Diplegia: paralysis of corresponding parts on both sides of the body.

Encephalitis: an inflammation of the brain.

Epidural hematoma: a head injury that causes blood to accumulate between the dura mater (the outer layer of membrane that covers the brain and spinal cord) and the skull.

Epilepsy: transient electrical disturbances in the brain that cause a temporary loss of speech or motor abilities, characterized by episodes of impairment or unconsciousness.

Headache: a general term for pain in the head. Migraine, cluster, and tension are all different types of headaches with differing symptoms.

Hemiplegia: paralysis that affects only one side of the body; also called hemiparesis.

Hemorrhage: the escape of blood from the vessels.

Huntington's chorea: a rare inherited disease of the central nervous system, with typical onset between 30 and 50 years of age, characterized by progressive dementia, abnormal posture, and involuntary movements.

Meningitis: an inflammation of the meninges (membranes) covering the brain and spinal cord.

Migraine: alternating vasoconstriction and vasodilation of the cerebral blood vessels, resulting in throbbing headache pain, double vision, sensitivity to light and noise, and other cerebral disturbances.

Monoplegia: paralysis that affects a single limb.

Myelitis: an inflammation of the spinal cord or bone marrow.

Paraplegia: paralysis of the legs and the lower part of the body.

Parkinson's disease: a progressive neurologic disease that begins with tremors and movement difficulties and eventually ends in dementia.

Quadriplegia: paralysis of all four limbs caused by stroke or a transection high in the spinal cord.

Residual ischemia neurological deficit: a particular lack of ability or activity that does not return after a stroke.

Reversible neurologic deficit: a lack of ability or activity that usually is reversed within 2 weeks of a stroke.

Schizophrenia: a mental disorder characterized by a disassociation from reality, including, but not limited to, delusions and hallucinations.

Seizure: a sudden onset of involuntary muscle contractions of the skeletal muscles, usually accompanied by a brief episode of unconsciousness. A petit mal seizure is brief in duration and causes a short period of loss of awareness and motor dysfunction. A grand mal seizure is more severe and results in loss of consciousness, incontinence, tongue-biting, and muscle contractions, followed by a state of confusion and lethargy. Also called a convulsion, fit, or attack.

Spinal cord injury: a lack of reflex or activity caused by trauma to the spinal cord. Cord contusion (bruising), cord concussion, cord compression, and cord laceration may result in temporary symptoms, whereas an incomplete or complete transection of the cord results in permanent injury.

Spinal shock: a temporary lack of reflex or activity below the level of a spinal cord injury.

Stroke: an impeded blood supply to some part of the brain, resulting in injury to brain tissue.

St. Vitus dance: a type of chorea that results from a strep infection followed by rheumatic fever.

Transient ischemic attack (TIA): a sudden attack that causes temporary loss of speech, movement, or other function caused by a temporary interruption of blood supply to the brain; normally less than 24 hours in duration; also called a mini-stroke.

Tumor: An abnormal mass of tissue resulting from uncontrolled progressive cell division. Tumors are either benign (harmless) or malignant (cancerous).

Here is a list of pathological conditions associated with the peripheral nervous system:

Bell's palsy: a paralysis of one side of the face caused by an impinged facial nerve; may be temporary and brought on by stress.

Benign paroxysmal positional vertigo (BPPV): a brief attack of vertigo that occurs only when the head is moved a certain way, caused by an inner ear (labyrinth) dysfunction.

Carpal tunnel syndrome: a compression of the median nerve in the wrist.

Compression: increasing pressure on a nerve or other structure.

Demyelination syndrome: the loss of a neuron's myelin sheath, with no damage to the axon or fiber pathways.

Diabetic neuropathy: a loss of sensation caused by damage to nerve cells due to poor circulation or hyperglycemia resulting from diabetes. Peripheral neuropathies usually affect the extremities; visceral neuropathies affect the cranial nerves and some of the internal organ systems, such as the GI tract and autonomic nervous system.

Entrapment: a constricted or distorted nerve.

Guillain–Barré syndrome: an acute infection of multiple nerves resulting in a loss of myelin and temporary loss of movement and sensation.

Herniated disc: an abnormal bulging of a vertebral disc from its normal place in the spinal column.

Herpes: a general term for any inflammatory skin disease caused by the herpes virus.

Herpes Simplex, type I: a virus that causes infections that are usually oral, although they can occur anywhere on the body.

Herpes Simplex, type II: a virus that causes infections that usually occur on the rectum and/or in the genital area, although they can occur anywhere on the body.

Ménière's disease: a recurring condition caused by a buildup of fluid in the inner ear, leading to episodes of deafness, vertigo, and ringing in the ears.

Multiple sclerosis (MS): a degenerative neurologic disease in which myelin is destroyed in the brain but not in the peripheral nerves.

Nerve root compression: abnormal pressure where a nerve emerges from the spinal cord.

Neuralgia: pain in the nerves.

Neuritis: inflammation of a nerve.

Neuropathy: a loss of feeling and/or function caused by degeneration in the distal end of a peripheral nerve.

Sciatica: a syndrome characterized by pain radiating from the lower back to the buttocks and down the lower extremity, usually caused by a prolapsed (displaced) disc; also used in a general way to describe any pain along the path of the sciatic nerve.

Shingles: a disease in adults that is caused by the same herpes virus that causes chicken pox in children; outbreaks arise from a latent virus in the spinal or cranial nerves.

Tarsal tunnel syndrome: a compression of the posterior tibial nerve resulting in pain or loss of sensation in the sole of the foot.

Thoracic outlet syndrome: a compression of the brachial plexus or subclavian artery.

Trigeminal neuralgia: a cranial nerve dysfunction that causes painful spasms in the lips, gums, cheeks, and chin areas of the face; also called tic douloureux.

Vertigo: an illusion of revolving through space or of space revolving around the person; often incorrectly used to describe dizziness.

Tips for Passing

Don't try to study when too many other things are distracting you. Multitasking is one thing; trying to do everything at once is something else. If you have small children who need attention, offer to trade babysitting duties with a classmate so you can both have uninterrupted study time. Let the answering machine get the phone. Turn the TV off, and put on some relaxing music. Make your atmosphere conducive to learning. Stand and stretch every 30 minutes or so.

Practice Questions

1. The nervous system includes these two separate systems
   a. The CNS and the PNF
   b. The CVS and the PNS
   c. The CNS and the PNS
   d. The CIS and PNF

2. The autonomic nervous system is part of the
   a. Collating nervous system
   b. Enteric nervous system
   c. Peripheral nervous system
   d. Central nervous system

3. The study of the nervous system is called
   a. Nerfology
   b. Neurology
   c. Nephrology
   d. Craniology

4. Neurotransmitters are
   a. Chemical messengers
   b. Short hairs that move the neurons
   c. Flagella
   d. Prokaryotes

5. The two ends of a neuron are called the
   a. Axis and the dendrite
   b. Axon and the dentine
   c. Axon and the dendrite
   d. Axis and the glia

6. The space between two cells is called the
   a. Borland gap
   b. Axolemma
   c. Renshaw opening
   d. Synapse

7. Dopamine is
   a. A chemical neurotransmitter
   b. A hormone
   c. Both a neurotransmitter and a hormone
   d. Neither a neurotransmitter nor a hormone

Affirmation

If I exercise my memory, it will serve me when I need it.

8. The myelin sheath is a layer of _____ surrounding the neuron.
   a. Insulation
   b. Infiltration
   c. Glial cells
   d. ATP

9. There are two main types of cells in the nervous tissue:
   a. Neurons and Golgi cells
   b. Spine cells and neurons
   c. Protons and glial cells
   d. Neurons and glial cells

10. _____ is a natural opiate produced by the brain to diminish pain.
   a. Endocrine
   b. Seratonin
   c. Endorphin
   d. Melatonin

CHAPTER 11

The Brain and Spinal Cord

The trick is to keep an open mind, without it being so open your brain falls out.

—CAMILLA CRACHIOLLO

HIGHLIGHTS

The brain, spinal cord, cranial nerves, and spinal nerves comprise the nervous system. The two most important structures of the nervous system are the brain and spinal cord. Chapter 10 covered the nervous system in general; this chapter focuses on the brain and spinal cord.

To borrow from computer language, the brain is the basic "central processing unit" of the body. It is estimated that the human brain contains more than 100 billion neurons. The center of our intellect, our ego, our emotions, our behavior, and our memory, the typical adult brain weighs 3 to 4 pounds.

The **brain** is composed of four main parts: the brainstem, the cerebellum, the diencephalon, and the cerebrum. The **brainstem** is the lowest part of the brain that integrates with the spinal cord. It consists of the medulla oblongata, the midbrain, and the pons. Cardiac and respiratory functions are regulated in the **medulla oblongata.** The **midbrain** is the top of the brainstem and regulates unconscious bodily functions. The **pons** contains a respiratory control center. The **cerebellum** helps maintain the body's sense of balance and muscle tone. The **diencephalon** relays information about sensation and motion, and it houses the **thalamus,** the **hypothalamus,** the **subthalamus,** and the **epithalamus.** The structures in the diencephalon are also believed to be involved in the body's emotional state. The **cerebrum** is the processing center for thought and higher reasoning.

The brain has three main functional areas: the sensory areas, which receive and interpret stimuli; the motor areas, which initiate movement; and the association areas, which facilitate more complex functions, such as intelligence, reasoning, and emotion. The brain is also divided into four lobes, the frontal, temporal, parietal, and occipital, which are separated by deep grooves known as sulci (singular, sulcus). The lobes and some of the major structures of the brain are shown in Figure 11.1.

The **sensory areas** include the primary somatosensory area, as well as the primary visual, auditory, gustatory, and olfactory areas. The primary somatosensory area, located in the **parietal lobe,** receives nerve impulses for the basic sensations of touch, pain, temperature, and proprioception, the self-regulation of posture and movement based on stimuli and responses. The **visual areas** receive impulses that convey visual information and process it into the images we see. The **auditory areas** receive impulses that help us to interpret sound, the **gustatory areas** receive information for taste, and the **olfactory areas** receive information for the sense of smell. There is some overlap among function in different areas of the brain. The **temporal lobe** contains auditory and receptive areas. The **occipital lobe** is the site of visual interpretation.

The **motor areas** include the primary motor area and Broca's speech area. The **primary motor area,** located in the **frontal lobe,** is subdivided into regions that control voluntary muscle movement in the different parts of the body. **Broca's speech area** controls the production of speech, with the assistance of several sensory, motor, and association areas of the **cerebral cortex,** the outer portion of the brain where thought processes take place.

The **association areas** of the brain include some motor and sensory areas as well, and they are interconnected through a system of association tracts (imagine the side streets in a neighborhood). Without the association areas, each experience or stimulus would be new every time. The association areas allow us to assimilate memories and enable us to compare each new experience with past experience. The **somatosensory**

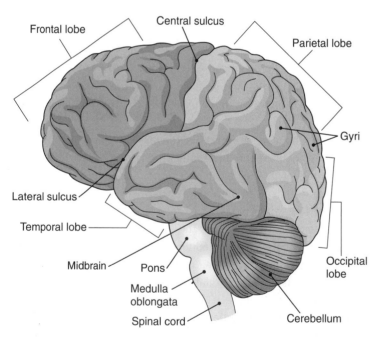

FIGURE 11.1
The external surface of the brain, showing the main parts and some lobes of the cerebrum. (Reprinted with permission from Cohen BJ. Medical Terminology: An Illustrated Guide, 4th ed. Philadelphia: Lippincott Williams & Wilkins; 2003. Fig. 17.3.)

association area interprets and integrates sensory information that comes into the body, and it is also the storehouse of past sensory experience; it is what helps you remember the smell of mom's apple pie or your favorite fragrance. The **visual association area** receives impulses and enables you to recognize things you have seen before and evaluate what action to take based on what you have seen. The **auditory association area** receives sound impulses and decides whether they are music, noise, or speech and enables you to recognize your favorite song. **Wernicke's area** (also called the **posterior language area**) interprets speech through the recognition of spoken words.

The **common integrative area (CIA)** receives impulses from all the areas and assimilates what it receives. The CIA is where our thoughts are formed and emotions arise that are based on past experiences. It is where everything comes together for us. The **premotor area** controls learned, intentional movements. My typing on this page is controlled by the premotor area. Your turning of the page is controlled by the premotor area. The **frontal eye field area** controls voluntary scanning movements of the eyes, such as when you are reading. The language areas receive signals from Broca's area and pass them to the appropriate mouth and throat muscles to make speech happen.

The cerebrum is divided into equal left and right **cerebral hemispheres.** The **limbic system** is a collection of structures in the brain located in a horseshoe-like rim of the cortices surrounding the junction between the diencephalon and each cerebral hemisphere. It consists of the **hippocampus,** the **amygdala,** the **fornicate gyrus,** and interconnecting structures. The limbic system is considered the mood center of the brain and is also involved in the regulation of the endocrine system and the autonomic nervous system.

Twelve pairs of cranial nerves arise from the underside of the brain; they are specialized sensory nerves, general sensory nerves, and nerves that are involved in both voluntary and involuntary movement (Table 11.1). Nerves also arise in 31 pairs from the **spinal cord,** which extends from the medulla oblongata to the second lumbar vertebra. The normal human body has eight pairs of **cervical nerves,** 12 pairs of **thoracic nerves,** five pairs of **lumbar nerves,** five pairs of **sacral nerves,** and one pair of **coccygeal nerves.**

The **meninges** are three connective tissue layers or membranes that cover the entire brain (cranial meninges) and spinal cord (spinal meninges). The outermost layer of the meninges is termed the **dura mater** (from Latin, meaning "tough mother"). The dura mater covers the entire brain and spinal cord down to S2, where it is closed on the end. The spinal cord is further protected by the space between the dura mater and the vertebrae, a fatty cushioned area called the **epidural space.** The middle layer of the meninges is called the **arachnoid,** because the delicate arrangement of collagen and elastic fibers resembles a spider's web. Between the dura matter and the arachnoid is an area called the **subdural space.** The third layer is called the **pia mater** ("delicate mother"). Between the arachnoid and the pia mater is an area called the **subarachnoid space.** The pia mater thickens into triangular processes called **denticulate ligaments.**

Chapter 12, on the craniosacral system, contains more information on the brain and spinal cord.

WHAT YOU NEED TO KNOW

Amygdala: a small almond-shaped brain structure that arouses nonverbal expressions of negative emotions, such as sweaty palms, dry mouth, and tense facial expressions.

TABLE 11.1 Table Listing the Cranial Nerves, Their Axons, and Important Function

Nerve Number and Name	Primary Functions
I. Olfactory	Sensation of smell
II. Optic	Sensation of Vision
III. Oculomotor	Eye and eyelid movements; control of pupil size
IV. Trochlear	Eye movements
V. Trigeminal	Sensation of touch to the face; movement of chewing muscles
VI. Abducens	Eye movement
VII. Facial	Movement of muscles of facial expression; sensation of taste in front of tongue
VIII. Auditory-vestibular	Sensations of hearing and balance
IX. Glossopharyngeal	Movement of throat muscles; control of the salivary glands; sensation of taste in back of tongue; detection of blood pressure changes
X. Vagus	Control of the heart, lungs, and abdominal organs; sensations of pain associated with internal organs; movement of throat muscles
XI. Spinal accessory	Movement of throat and neck muscles
XII. Hypoglossal	Movement of tongue

Arachnoid villi: long tubules extending from the arachnoid that serve as one-way valves for cerebrospinal fluid to exit the brain and enter the bloodstream.

Association fibers: brain fibers in the cerebral cortex that are involved in processing, but not in the strict sense of motor or sensory.

Basal ganglia: paired clusters of cell bodies that make up the central gray matter in each cerebral hemisphere; they work together with the cerebral cortex to refine movements, feelings, and thoughts.

Blood–brain barrier (BBB): a protective layer of blood vessels and glial cells that keep most substances from penetrating through to the brain from the bloodstream.

Brainstem: the lowest part of the brain; refers collectively to the medulla oblongata, the midbrain, and the pons.

Cauda equina: the root of all nerves that occur below L1; the lower end of the spinal cord.

Central canal: a cavity that is the location of the spinal cord.

Cerebellum: part of the back brain, primarily concerned with movement, muscle tone, and balance.

Cerebral aqueduct: a canal in the midbrain that connects the third and fourth ventricles.

Cerebral cortex: the outer portion of the brain where thought processes take place.

Cerebrospinal fluid (CSF): a clear, colorless fluid, composed mostly of glucose and protein, that surrounds the brain and spinal cord and fills the ventricles of the brain and the central canal of the spinal cord; provides protection and nutrients.

Cerebrum: the largest and most forward (anterior) portion of the brain; functions include higher cognitive functions.

Epithalamus: the dorsal posterior section of the diencephalon.

Falx cerebelli: a short process of the dura mater extending from the occipital crest.

Falx cerebri: a fold of the dura mater located between the two cerebral hemispheres in the longitudinal fissure (deep fold).

Gyrus: one of the rounded ridges (gyri) associated with the surface of the cerebrum.

Hippocampus: the part of the brain thought to be associated with long-term memory.

Hypothalamus: the part of the brain that secretes chemicals that help regulate body temperature, thirst, hunger, water balance, and sexual function; also closely connected with emotional activity and sleep; functions as the center for the integration of hormonal and autonomic nervous activity.

Interventricular foramina: a short slit-like passage that connects the third ventricle area of the brain to the lateral ventricles.

Limbic system: a brain area consisting of the amygdala, the hypothalamus, and other structures that affect the endocrine system and autonomic motor system; the limbic system also affects moods and motivational states.

Lumbar enlargement: an expanded region of the spinal cord that starts at T10 and is thickest at the last thoracic vertebra.

Medulla oblongata: the lowest division of the brainstem, immediately above the spinal cord; involved in cardiac and respiratory functions.

Mesencephalon: the midbrain.

Olfactory bulb: the egg-shaped body from which the olfactory (smell) nerves extend.

Olive: an olive-shaped prominence on either side of the medulla oblongata.

Pineal gland: a small flat gland that produces melatonin and serotonin.

Plexus: a network of nerves.

Pons: one of the structures located in the lower brainstem just above the spinal cord; acts as a major pathway for motor and sensory information between the body and higher-level brain functioning.

Posterior root: the sensory root of a spinal nerve.

Sulcus: a groove on the surface of the cerebrum, lying between adjacent gyri.

Tentorium cerebelli: a fold of the dura mater that separates the cerebrum from the cerebellum.

Thalamus: two large ovoid masses composed mostly of gray matter, situated on either side of the third ventricle.

Ventricle: a hollow space in the central brain (also applies to a hollow space in other organs).

PATHOLOGY OF THE BRAIN AND SPINAL CORD

Some pathological conditions that may affect the brain and spinal cord are not caused by or directly related to the nervous system. Spinal cord injuries and other conditions that do affect the nervous system have already been defined in Chapter 10.

Many conditions that affect the brain involve chemical imbalances that alter emotional and mental states, such as affective and anxiety disorders, sleep disorders, perceptual anomalies like deafness or blindness, disorders of development, and degenerative disorders. **Tumors** (defined in Chapter 10) may affect the brain without direct involvement of the nervous system on the whole. Even a brain tumor that is benign can cause compression severe enough to damage adjacent tissues and create neurological problems. A **glioma** is the most serious type of brain tumor, a fast-growing tumor that **metastasizes** or spreads, invading surrounding tissue and destroying healthy cells in its path. Tumors may also appear on or near the spinal cord, causing interference with nerve function. This can cause constant pain, loss of sensation, and/or the loss of many abilities—everything from bladder and bowel control to the ability to control movements, and even paralysis.

Some developmental disorders are caused by the mother and/or fetus being exposed to dangerous toxins, as in **fetal alcohol syndrome,** or to abnormalities caused by a drug that is contraindicated for pregnant mothers. During the 1960s, many children were born with deformities because their mothers took thalidomide, a drug that was prescribed for morning sickness.

Inherited metabolic disorders can also cause brain damage or impede normal development. There are more than 100 such disorders. **Tay–Sachs disease,** which mainly affects children of Eastern European Jewish descent, causes the brain to swell and damage itself against the insides of the skull. Children with Tay–Sachs have no chance of a normal life and can expect to survive only a few years at most. **Phenylketonuria (PKU)** is another inherited metabolic disorder caused by the absence of a necessary enzyme. PKU results in profound mental retardation from abnormal brain development.

Depression, anxiety, and some of the other disorders that were mentioned in Chapter 10 and that are caused by direct neurological involvement deserve further explanation. Common depression may be a temporary state of sadness, such as grief over the death of a loved one or some other tangible event, but **clinical depression** persists for more than 2 weeks and involves extreme fatigue, change of habits and personality, and possibly suicidal thoughts. Chronically depressed people cannot name a reason for their despair. Current theories are that levels of the neurotransmitters norepinephrine and serotonin cause depression. **Bipolar disorder** results in periods of depression followed by periods of **mania,** erratic behavior that is the opposite of depression. A manic person talks fast (too fast for their thinking), has unusual enthusiasm and, often, euphoric behavior, and may be delusional in some cases.

Listed are some other brain and spinal disorders:

Arteriovenous malformation: a condition in which blood in the brain is shunted directly from the arteries to the veins, bypassing the capillaries, resulting in an area that lacks oxygen. Symptoms (headache, seizures) appear after age 30.

Autism: a brain disorder of unknown origin causing developmental problems in children in the areas of speech, behavior, and social skills.

Brain abscess: a pus-filled cavity caused by a bacterial infection.

Cerebral trauma: a brain injury.

Coma: a prolonged state of deep unconsciousness as a result of trauma or illness.

Delirium: an acute mental disorder that affects the ability to reason and causes speech impairment and other cerebral dysfunctions; organic in cause and often reversible.

Dementia pugilistica: the cumulative effects of being hit on the head numerous times; also known as the "punch drunk" and "boxer's affliction."

Down syndrome: mental retardation caused by the possession of an extra chromosome 21.

Hydrocephalus: abnormally increased CSF surrounding the brain ("water on the brain").

Insomnia: an inability to sleep.

Lethargy: abnormal drowsiness or stupor.

Narcolepsy: a sleep disorder characterized by an inability to stay awake; consists of sudden bouts of sleeping at inappropriate times and inability to sleep at night.

Sleep apnea: a temporary interruption in breathing that occurs during sleep.

Spina bifida: a birth defect in which the vertebral arch (the posterior projection from the body of the vertebra) fails to close around the spinal cord and meninges.

Substance-related disorders: dysfunctions that may include mood disturbances, sleep disturbances, sexual dysfunction, withdrawal delirium, intoxification, and dementia, caused by drug abuse or side effects of medication or toxic exposure.

 Tips for Passing

Thinking of nerve impulses as a telephone line is a very good idea. There are countless *visual* keys you can use to help yourself remember all the facts. If the telephone image doesn't work for you, think of a wide receiver (the dendrites) catching a pass and running down the field (the axons), or whatever other visual works for you. Rationalize to yourself *right now* that it behooves you, as a massage therapist, to know the nerves and where they go, and start memorizing them. You will appear more knowledgeable to a client, when she mentions she can't extend her wrist, if you can point out the radial nerve on your chart as the nerve involved in that movement (being careful, of course, not to make a diagnosis). This is not just a tip for passing the NCE; it's a tip for being an effective massage therapist. Nerves are usually involved in loss of sensation or loss of the ability to make a particular movement. As you mature into a more experienced massage therapist, you will not just "work on their arm." You will perform an assessment to see what motion can't be made or made without pain, and then isolate the muscle(s) and/or nerve(s) involved in those movements, and work from there.

Practice Questions

1. It is estimated that the human brain contains _____ neurons.
   a. Approximately 1 million
   b. Approximately 10,000
   c. Approximately 10 million
   d. Approximately 100 billion

2. Intelligence, reasoning, and emotion are facilitated in the _____ area of the brain.
   a. Motor
   b. Sensory

Affirmation

I have confidence in myself and in my ability to pass the test.

    c. Association

    d. Somatic

3. Wernicke's area of the brain

    a. Allows recognition of colors

    b. Interprets speech

    c. Causes sinuses to drain

    d. Controls intentional movements

4. There are _____ pairs of nerves arising from the spinal cord.

    a. 31

    b. 32

    c. 33

    d. 34

5. The meninges include

    a. Spinal and cranial meninges

    b. Cervical and abdominal meninges

    c. Cervical and cranial meninges

    d. Spinal and thoracic meninges

6. Past sensory experiences are stored in the

    a. Broca's area

    b. Arachnoid villi

    c. Motor area

    d. Somatosensory association area

7. The part of the brain associated with long-term memory is the

    a. Hypothalamus

    b. Medulla oblongata

    c. Hippocampus

    d. Pons

8. Melatonin and serotonin are produced in the

    a. Pituitary gland

    b. Thyroid gland

    c. Sebaceous gland

    d. Pineal gland

9. The protective layer that keeps most substances from penetrating through to the brain from the blood is the

    a. CAT

    b. CIA

    c. BBB

    d. AAL

10. The long tubules extending from the arachnoid and pia mater that act as one-way valves for the cerebrospinal fluid are the

    a. Erector pili

    b. Intake channels

    c. Arachnoid villi

    d. Pia mater

The Craniosacral System

Everything's in the mind. That's where it all starts. Knowing what you want is the first step toward getting it.

—MAE WEST

HIGHLIGHTS

Some massage schools do not address the craniosacral system as a separate system or a form of bodywork. If that was the case at your school, you may want to read *Your Inner Physician and You,* a short paperback by Dr. John Upledger, an osteopathic physician, for a simple explanation. This chapter addresses craniosacral bodywork as well as the structures and functions of the system because the National Board does treat it as a separate system. Many Western physicians still do not acknowledge a separate craniosacral system. Medical schools still teach that the skull bones are fused and don't move. Upledger and others who teach the craniosacral modalities state the opposite—that the skull bones do move and if they don't, it is because the sutures (the fibrous joints of the skull) are constricted and need to be loosened. The sutures, along with the major bones and fontanels (soft spots), are shown in Figure 12.1.

Osteopathy is a branch of medicine based on the premise that the body is a vital organism capable of healing itself when conditions are optimum and correct nutrition is followed. Osteopathy often encompasses chiropractic, massage therapy, and other complementary forms of health care, including craniosacral therapy. Whereas Upledger is most widely known for his method of craniosacral therapy today, his work is based on the theories of William Sutherland, also a Doctor of Osteopathy. Sutherland was the first to declare the craniosacral as a separately functioning system with its own rhythm and to observe that cranial bones do move. **Craniosacral rhythm** is the rhythmic rise and fall of the craniosacral fluid. Upledger expanded on Sutherland's

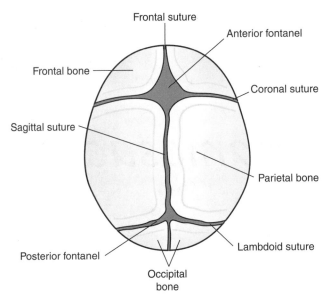

FIGURE 12.1
Sutures and fontanels of the skull. (Reprinted with permission from Pilliteri A. Maternal and Child Nursing, 4th ed. Philadelphia: Lippincott, Williams & Wilkins; 2003. Fig. 52.1.)

work to develop his "pressurestat" theory, the idea that cerebrospinal fluid is produced at a much faster rate than it is reabsorbed and that the craniosacral rhythm is caused by some type of homeostatic regulation. The rate of the craniosacral system is normally 6 to 8 beats per minute, according to Upledger's teaching. Some proponents state the craniosacral rate as high as 10 to 14 beats per minute. Other modalities that address the system include cranial therapy, biocranial therapy, craniopathy, and sacral-occipital technique. The craniosacral system is shown in Figure 12.2.

Some of the terms from Chapters 10 and 11 are repeated here for clarification of their relation to the craniosacral system. The structures of the **craniosacral system** are the three-layered membrane system called the **meninges;** the tissues in the four **ventricles** of the brain where the cerebrospinal fluid is produced (referred to as the **choroid plexus**); the **cerebrospinal fluid (CSF);** and nerves that control the **parasympathetic** division of the **autonomic nervous system (ANS).** The parasympathetic nerves are located in the cranial and sacral regions of the spinal cord; hence, the term *craniosacral.* The parasympathetic system slows the heart rate, increases glandular and intestinal activity, and relaxes the sphincter muscles. The parasympathetic nervous system is sometimes referred to as "rest and digest" and has the opposite actions of the sympathetic nervous system, which is often referred to as the "fight-or-flight" system.

The innermost layer of the meninges is the **pia mater** ("delicate mother"). This membrane, with lots of blood vessels, totally encompasses the brain and the spinal cord. The middle layer is the **arachnoid,** reinforced by soft fibers arranged like a cobweb. The **dura mater** ("tough mother") is the outermost membrane protecting the brain and spinal cord. The dura mater is made up of two distinct layers. The outer layer, the **periosteal layer,** attaches to the **periosteum** of the skull bones. The inner layer, the **meningeal layer,** is normally fused to the outer layer with some spaces in between for blood vessels and sinus cavities.

Most of our organs have dual innervation, receiving nerve impulses from both sympathetic and parasympathetic neurons. Because of their opposing actions, when

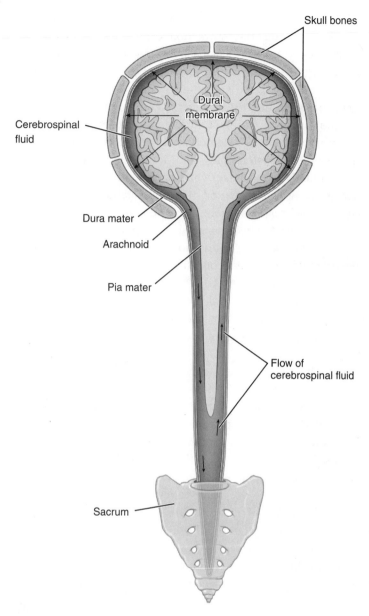

Skull bones

Dural membrane

Cerebrospinal fluid

Dura mater

Arachnoid

Pia mater

Flow of cerebrospinal fluid

Sacrum

FIGURE 12.2
The craniosacral system of the CSF and dural membrane.

nerve impulses direct something to speed up activity in one system, something will slow down in the other system. However, although the sympathetic nervous system is known as the fight-or-flight system, when extreme fear takes over, the parasympathetic nervous system kicks in. When confronted with sheer terror, we may lose control of normal bowel or bladder function because of parasympathetic involvement.

The cerebrospinal fluid contains glucose and protein and flows through the meninges covering the brain and the spinal cord. The axons of the parasympathetic **preganglionic neurons** are referred to as the **craniosacral parasympathetic outflow.** They extend from the central nervous system to a **terminal ganglion** in an innervated organ.

The **craniosacral nerves** are involved in many various actions in different parts of the body. In the eyes, the nerves affect the secretion of tears, the contraction of the pupils, and the contraction of the iris for close-up vision. In the digestive system, the craniosacral nerves affect the contraction of the gallbladder and ducts for increased secretion of bile, the synthesis of glycogen (storage form of glucose), the secretion of bile from the liver, the secretion of gastric juices in the stomach, and increased salivary production. They also relax the sphincter muscles of the digestive system and the urinary system. In the circulatory system, the craniosacral nerves affect a decrease in the heart rate and vasoconstriction of the heart arterioles. In the reproductive system, the craniosacral nerves effect the erection of the clitoris in females and the penis in males. In the respiratory system, they contract the lungs and the bronchial muscles.

The acronym SLUDD might help you remember the functions of the parasympathetic system: salivation, lacrimation (tears), urination, digestion, and defecation. These are all "increase" responses. The parasympathetic nervous system also controls the decrease of the heart rate, constriction of the airways, and constriction of the pupils. From these various increases and decreases, you can understand how the rhythm of the craniosacral system collectively maintains the rhythm of many different body functions.

Craniosacral therapy is a form of bodywork aimed at releasing constrictions that inhibit the free flow of the CSF. According to Upledger, anything that interferes with the ability of the dura mater to accommodate the rhythmically fluctuating fluid pressures and volumes is a potential trouble source. A tear in the membrane opens the body to the possibility of infection. A constriction in the membrane can cause interference with the transmission of nerve impulses, which can lead to a multitude of problems—from headaches to menstrual pain to lack of energy, even to hormonal imbalances. The craniosacral therapist "tunes in" to the rhythm of the CSF and learns to detect blockages or other deviations that may be restricting the normal flow of fluid.

In my own training in craniosacral therapy, we were first taught how to feel the rhythm by holding the feet, palms placed under the heel and fingertips lightly resting just above the medial malleolus. That exercise was followed by several techniques that can be easily incorporated into massage sessions without having to be a craniosacral expert. Releasing the occiput (the back of the head) and releasing the sacrum are two of the most useful techniques.

Myofascial "unwinding" is a technique of holding an area with both hands and allowing the tissue to go where it wants to go. This simple action releases restrictions in the fascia that are often nothing more than symptomatic of poor body-use habits. Gentle pulling, twisting, and turning relax the connective tissue and allow it to reach a discernible instant of release, known as the **still point.** The practitioner also looks for resistances and blockages in bones, membranes, tissues, and fluids of the body that might also be affecting energy flow and physiological function. The goal of the therapist is to facilitate the body's own potential for physical release and emotional clearing, bringing itself back into balance. Just being aware of the energy flow and resistances, and using the lightest touch with the intention of restoring balance, is often enough to stimulate release on one or many levels—whether physical, emotional, or energetic. Most of the craniosacral modalities recommend using touch equivalent in pressure to a nickel resting on the skin.

Craniosacral bodywork does contain an emotional component. The premise is that each trauma is recorded in the body and, unless released, stays there. Every scare we've ever experienced is there, along with every fall we've ever taken, every broken heart, and every bumped knee, recorded in our tissues and just waiting to be released. Craniosacral therapy is aimed at releasing perpetuated patterns of muscle tension, pain, and stress and replacing them with awareness.

Craniosacral is a very gentle yet powerful modality that brings about deep relaxation. It is usually performed with the client fully clothed. The practitioner's touch is very subtle, but clients report feeling a sense of release in deep tissue and relief of long-held pain. In addition to the release of physical tension and the emotional release experienced by many clients, craniosacral practitioners believe that all manner of headaches, CNS disorders, temporomandibular joint syndrome, scoliosis, connective tissue diseases, and many more conditions can be effectively treated using craniosacral therapy.

Whether you personally choose to believe in the efficacy of craniosacral therapy, you still need to be familiar with the anatomy and physiology of the system. This is not a tip for passing the examination but a tip for educating yourself as a therapist. Make it a point to seek out therapists who practice modalities that you don't know and experience them for yourself. Not only will you be receiving the therapeutic value of the session but also will you take away a few tricks to add to your repertoire. Think of it as continuing your education while you're taking care of yourself.

WHAT YOU NEED TO KNOW

The definitions in Chapters 10 and 11 should be studied in addition to those listed below.

Arachnoid: the middle layer of the three meninges; made of collagen and elastic fibers that resemble a spider's web, hence the name.

Cranial parasympathetic outflow: axons of parasympathetic preganglionic neurons extending from the brain in four cranial nerves.

Dural membrane: another term for meninges; the three-layered membrane covering the brain and spinal cord.

Dura mater: the outer layer of the meninges; from Latin for "tough mother."

Epidural space: the space between the dura mater and the wall of the vertebral canal.

Pia mater: the tender innermost layer of the meninges, from Latin for "delicate mother."

Sacral parasympathetic outflow: axons of parasympathetic preganglionic neurons extending from the brain in the anterior roots of the second through the fourth sacral nerves.

Subdural space: the layer between the dura mater and the arachnoid containing interstitial fluid.

PATHOLOGY OF THE CRANIOSACRAL SYSTEM

Pathological conditions involving the craniosacral system are included in Chapters 10 and 11. Compressed nerves are often the focus of craniosacral therapists, who believe that almost any condition in the body can be related to restrictions in the flow of CSF and improved by craniosacral therapy—a view that many doctors dismiss.

Tips for Passing

Not enough hours in the day? Try setting your alarm to get up an hour or a half-hour earlier and use that time to study. The house is quiet, the family is still asleep, and you can have a nice cup of coffee or tea and study undisturbed. Your memory will likely be a little sharper than it is after a stressful day of work, homemaking, and other obligations.

Practice Questions

1. Cerebrospinal fluid contains
   a. Proteins and carbohydrates
   b. Vitamins and minerals
   c. Glucose and protein
   d. Nitrogen and hydrogen

2. The craniosacral system includes
   a. Nerves that control the parasympathetic division of the ANS
   b. Only the nerves that go to the head
   c. Nerves located in the thoracic area
   d. None of the above

3. The membrane that covers the brain and the spinal cord has _____ layers.
   a. 1
   b. 2
   c. 3
   d. 4

4. Dura mater means
   a. Dead mother
   b. Big mother
   c. Tough mother
   d. Small mother

5. The craniosacral nerves are involved in
   a. The secretion of bile
   b. Relaxing sphincter muscles
   c. The erection of the sex organs
   d. All of the above

6. The arachnoid is made of
   a. Tendons and ligaments
   b. Collagen and elastic fibers
   c. Enzymes and protein
   d. Hyaline cartilage

7. Craniosacral rhythm refers to
   a. The time it takes for a nerve impulse to travel from the head to the sacrum
   b. The time in between each breath
   c. The rise and fall of the cerebrospinal fluid
   d. The movement of gas through the bowels

8. The pia mater is the _____ dural membrane.
   a. Outer
   b. Inner
   c. Middle
   d. None of the above

9. The subdural space contains
   a. Lymph
   b. Interstitial fluid
   c. Blood
   d. Nitrogenous waste

10. The epidural space is between the
    a. Dura mater and the pia mater
    b. Dura mater and the wall of the vertebral canal
    c. Brain and the subdural space
    d. Dura mater and the occipital ridge

CHAPTER 13

The Endocrine System

Memory is the only way home.

—TERRY TEMPEST WILLIAMS

HIGHLIGHTS

The study of the endocrine system and related diseases and disorders is known as **endocrinology.** The structures of the endocrine system are various **glands** and other hormone-producing organs, such as the kidneys and the stomach. Glands are made up of specialized groups of cells that produce and secrete **hormones** to regulate many body functions. The glands of the endocrine system release hormones directly into the bloodstream, where they act as chemical messengers of the body; a number of hormones also function as **neurotransmitters** in the nervous system. The endocrine glands are listed in Table 13.1, along with their location, secretions, and functions.

Each gland responds to changes in the body, including changes in the makeup of blood, by secreting **hormone.** Hormones act as a signal to specific areas of the body that work to correct the change. Hormones affect only those target cells that are genetically programmed to receive and respond to that particular hormone.

Hormones, just like synthetic hormones or other drugs, have a **half-life,** a point in time in which the concentration is half of what it was at full concentration in the fluid or blood. In a **negative-feedback system,** the chemicals can act at an earlier stage to prohibit their own development as part of the regulatory process of the endocrine system as a whole. Although hormones are produced primarily by the endocrine glands, there are other organs of the body that also produce and release hormones: the brain, lungs, heart, kidneys, liver, and skin. **Exocrine glands** are glands that secrete through a duct, such as **sweat glands** or the **mammary glands.**

TABLE 13.1 Endocrine Glands

Endocrine Gland	Location	Secretions	Functions
Anterior pituitary	Anterior half of gland located at base of brain in depression (fossa) of sphenoid bone, in front of occipital in base of skull	Thyroid-stimulating hormone (TSH)	Stimulates secretions from thyroid gland
		Adrenocorticotropic hormone (ACTH)	Stimulates secretion from adrenal cortex
		Follicle-stimulating hormone (FSH)	Initiates growth of ovarian follicle; stimulates secretion of estrogen in females and sperm production in males
		Luteinizing hormone (LH)	Causes ovulation; secretion of progesterone and testosterone
		Melanocyte-stimulating hormone (MSH)	Affects skin pigmentation
		Human growth hormone (HGH)	Influences growth
		Prolectin (lactogenic hormone)	Stimulates breast development and milk production during pregnancy
Posterior pituitary	Posterior half of gland located at base of brain in depression (fossa) of sphenoid bone, in front of occipital in base of skull	Antidiuretic hormone (ADH)	Influences absorption of water by kidney tubules
		Oxytocin	Influences uterine contractions
Pineal gland	At back of third ventricle of brain	Melatonin	Exact function unknown; affects onset of puberty
		Serotonin	Acts as precursor to melatonin
Thyroid gland	In neck on both sides of trachea	Thyroxine Triiodothyronine	Regulates metabolism
		Calcitonin	Regulates calcium and phosphorus metabolism
Parathyroid glands	In region of thyroid gland	Parathyroid hormone (PTH)	Regulates calcium and phosporus metabolism
Pancreas (islets of Langerhans)	Inferior and posterior to stomach; islets of Langerhans are within pancreas	Insulin, glucagon, somatostatin	Regulates carbohydrate, fat, and protein metabolism
Thymus gland	Behind stenum in space between lungs	Thymosin	Regulates immune response
Adrenal gland	One above each kidney	Steroid hormones; glucocorticoids, mineral corticosteroids, androgens	Regulates carbohydrate metabolism and salt and water balance; some effect on sexual characteristics

continued

TABLE 13.1 Endocrine Glands (*Continued*)			
Endocrine Gland	**Location**	**Secretions**	**Functions**
		Epinephrine, norepinephrine	Affects sympathetic nervous system in stress response
Ovaries	One on either sides of uterus	Estrogen, progesterone	Responsible for development of female secondary sex characteristics and regulation of reproduction
Testes	In cavity of scrotum	Testosterone	Affects masculinization and reproduction

The tiny **pituitary gland,** which is the size of a pea, is often referred to as the "master gland" because it produces the hormones that control several other glands. It is also called the **hypophysis.** The pituitary is divided into two lobes. The **anterior lobe** produces **human growth hormone (HGH)** and regulates the thyroid, the reproductive glands, and the adrenal glands. HGH stimulates the liver to produce an insulin-like substance that supports the growth of the musculoskeletal system. The anterior lobe also secretes **adrenocorticotropic hormone (ATCH),** which maintains the adrenal cortex, and **thyroid-stimulating hormone (TSH).** In women, the anterior lobe secretes **follicle-stimulating hormone (FSH),** which stimulates the release of eggs and the release of estrogen. **Luteinizing hormone (LH)** acts with FSH to stimulate the release of sex hormones. Along with **prolactin,** another protein, these hormones are collectively known as the **anterior pituitary hormones.** The **posterior lobe** of the pituitary controls the balance of water in the body through **antidiuretic hormone (ADH)** and also secretes the hormone **oxytocin,** which causes the uterus to contract during labor.

The two **adrenal glands** are located one on top of each kidney and produce many hormones that are known as **steroids.** The **adrenal cortex,** the outer part of the glands, produces hormones called **corticosteroids,** which help maintain the balance of salt and water in the body; they aid the immune system, the reproductive system, and help maintain metabolism. **Glucocorticoids,** such as **cortisol,** have powerful effects on carbohydrate, fat, and protein metabolism. The **adrenal medulla,** the inner part of the adrenal gland, produces hormones such as adrenaline (also referred to as epinephrine) known as **catecholamines,** which help regulate the heart rate and blood pressure whenever the body is under stress, by mobilizing the body's fuel for use. The most important part of the adrenal glands is their involvement in helping the body respond to stress.

The **pineal gland,** located in the middle of the brain, helps regulate the body's wake–sleep cycle through the production of **melatonin.** Other hormones and neurotransmitters have also been identified in the pineal gland, including **serotonin, dopamine, histamine,** and **norepinephrine.** The **hypothalamus,** a section of the brain situated under the **thalamus,** secretes chemicals that help regulate metabolism by influencing the actions of the pituitary gland.

The **gonads,** the main source of sex hormones, are discussed thoroughly in Chapter 19 on the reproductive system. The primary sex hormones are **estrogen** and **progesterone** in females and **testosterone** in males. Sex hormones begin to be secreted around puberty and cause the development of secondary sex characteristics, such as breasts in females and facial hair in males, as well as menstruation and pregnancy in females and the production of sperm in males. **Relaxin** is a hormone produced in the blood of pregnant women that aids in muscle relaxation during childbirth.

The **thyroid gland** regulates the body's metabolism by controlling the rate at which the body's cells turn fuel (food) into energy. The body's **basal metabolic rate (BMR)** refers to the rate the body metabolizes when it is at a resting state, typically 12 hours after the last meal. Metabolic changes occur in response to eating, temperature, stress, illness, and many other things.

The **parathyroid glands** are four small structures attached to the thyroid. The level of calcium in the body is regulated by the secretion of **parathyroid hormone (PTH).** People with **hypoparathyroidism** produce too little of this hormone; people with **hyperparathyroidism** produce too much. **Hypoparathyroidism** is characterized by low blood calcium levels and causes muscle spasms, decreased metabolism, lethargy, sensitivity to cold, and menstrual problems. **Hyperparathyroidism** is characterized by too much calcium in the blood and causes increased metabolism, high blood pressure, and related symptoms.

The **pancreas** secretes **insulin, somatostatin,** and **glucagon,** which help maintain blood sugar levels and keep the body's fat and protein metabolism regulated. Within the pancreas, the **islets of Langerhans** are cell groups that produce insulin and glucagons. The islets, along with nerves and mucus of the gastrointestinal tract, posterior pituitary, and hypothalamus, contain the hormone **somatostatin,** which inhibits gastric secretions and motility in the GI tract.

The **thymus gland** produces several substances and is involved in the differentiation of T cells—lymphocytes that are important to the body's immune system. **Thymopoietin** and **thymic factor** aid in **differentiation,** the process cells undergo as they mature. **Thymosin** is also vital to the body's immune function.

Other tissues of the body are also involved in hormone production; they are known as **tissue hormones. Histamines** are potent chemical agents that cause localized immune responses, such as a reaction to a bee sting or venomous snakebite. **Atrial natriuretic factor (ANF)** facilitates the release of excess sodium through the urine. **Erythropoietin** is a special growth hormone secreted by the kidneys that regulates the production of red blood cells in the bone marrow. **Insulin-like growth factor (IGF-1)** is a protein that is similar in structure to insulin and is involved with stimulating growth in bone and cartilage. **Gastrointestinal hormones** within the GI tract or digestive organs regulate the secretions of the GI tract. **Gastrin** is secreted whenever there is food in the stomach and during times of stress. **Secretin** inhibits the secretion of gastric acid while encouraging pancreatic, bile, and pepsin secretions. **Cholecystokinin (CKK)** facilitates the contractions of the gallbladder and pancreatic secretions. **Prostaglandins** are involved in many diverse functions of the body.

The **stress response**—also known as the **general adaptation syndrome, or GAS**—is a series of changes that occur in the body whenever we are under stress. Hormone levels can be affected not only by stress but also by infection or changes in the balance of fluid and minerals in the blood.

WHAT YOU NEED TO KNOW

Adrenal cortex: the outer part of the adrenal gland that inhibits inflammation through the production of cortisol; regulates minerals in the blood and produces sex hormones.

Adrenal gland: an endocrine gland located above the kidney. The adrenal glands help control heart rate and blood pressure and regulate the fight-or-flight stress response.

Adrenal medulla: the inner part of the adrenal gland that produces epinephrine and norepinephrine, hormones that are released in response to stress.

Adrenocorticotropic hormone (ACTH): an anterior pituitary hormone that maintains the adrenal cortex and stimulates the cortex to produce steroids.

Anterior pituitary gland: one of two lobes of the pituitary; produces human growth hormone and hormones that stimulate the thyroid, adrenals, and gonads.

Antidiuretic hormone (ADH): a posterior pituitary hormone that increases the reabsorption of water in the kidneys to decrease urine production.

Calcitonin: a thyroid hormone that controls the levels of calcium and phosphorous in the blood.

Cortisol: the main hormone produced by the adrenal glands; raises blood sugar level, promotes glycogen breakdown in the liver, and stimulates the change of proteins into carbohydrates.

Dopamine: a neurotransmitter that is usually activated by stress; acts to inhibit the transmission of nerve impulses.

Epidermal growth factor (EGF): promotes cell growth and specialization, is essential in embryo development, and important in wound healing; it is produced by many normal cell types and some tumors.

Epinephrine: an adrenal hormone that stimulates blood flow; also called adrenaline.

Estrogen: a sex hormone produced in the ovaries (the female gonads); regulates the menstrual cycle and the development of the female sexual organs and secondary sex characteristics.

Fibroblast growth factor: a hormone produced by many tissues that stimulates cell growth and the growth of new blood vessels.

Follicle-stimulating hormone (FSH): an anterior pituitary hormone that stimulates the production of sperm in males and the development of the follicle, a structure within the ovaries that produces eggs.

Gonads: glands that produce sex cells (also called gametes) and sex hormones. In males, the gonads are the testes, which produce testosterone. In females, the gonads are the ovaries, which produce estrogen and progesterone.

Human growth hormone (HGH): an anterior pituitary hormone that controls the growth of bones and soft tissues; involved in metabolizing fat in the body.

Insulin: a pancreatic hormone that lowers blood sugar levels by facilitating the uptake of glucose by the cells.

Luteinizing hormone (LH): an anterior pituitary hormone that promotes ovulation in females and stimulates testosterone production in males.

Melatonin: a hormone produced in the pineal gland, thought to be the regulator of the body's circadian rhythms, the 24-hour cycle of regularly recurring processes such as eating and sleeping.

Nerve growth factor: a hormone produced by a variety of tissues that facilitates the growth of the ganglia (nerve tissue) in embryos and the differentiation of neurons, and maintains the balance of the sympathetic nervous system.

Norepinephrine: a neurotransmitter that prepares the body for stress by regulating heart rate and oxygen delivery.

Ovary: the female gonad in which eggs (ova) are developed and released during ovulation.

Pancreas: a gland that secretes insulin and pancreatic enzymes that aid in the digestion of food.

Parathyroid gland: one of four tiny glands attached to (or buried within) the thyroid; secretes hormones that regulate blood calcium levels, which affect many bodily functions.

Pineal gland: a small gland in the midbrain where melatonin and serotonin are produced.

Pituitary gland: a pea-sized gland in the brain comprised of anterior and posterior lobes; called the "master gland" because it produces the hormones that control several other glands.

Platelet-derived growth factor: a hormone produced in the blood platelets that appears to facilitate the healing of wounds.

Posterior pituitary gland: one of the two lobes of the pituitary; produces ADH and the hormone oxytocin, which stimulates uterine contractions during childbirth as well as lactation.

Progesterone: a sex hormone; an antagonist of estrogen produced by the ovaries; prepares the uterus for the implantation of a fertilized egg and prevents miscarriage by preserving the uterine lining.

Testis: the male gonad (plural: testes).

Testosterone: a male sex hormone; regulates the production of sperm and causes the growth of male secondary sex characteristics.

Thymus: an organ located above the heart that produces T cells—specialized cells of the immune system.

Thyroid gland: located below the larynx; an endocrine gland that regulates metabolism.

PATHOLOGY OF THE ENDOCRINE SYSTEM

The pathology of the endocrine system can be categorized into conditions that are caused by malfunctions of the various glands or other hormone-producing organs. When regulatory processes fail, **hypersecretion,** an excessive production of hormone, or **hyposecretion,** a deficiency of hormone production, results. Some types of cancer produce hormone-like substances that can cause endocrine system problems. Sometimes the target cells of a particular substance malfunction and do not receive the necessary instruction to speed up or slow down production. This creates an **abnormal metabolic response** in the body, resulting in a pathological condition.

Acromegaly: a pituitary disorder in the adult caused by excessive amounts of growth hormone, characterized by overly large lips and nose, enlarged jawbones and forehead, and abnormally enlarged bones in the extremities.

Addison's disease: an endocrine disease resulting from hyposecretion of mineralocorticoids and glucocorticoids from the adrenal glands, which results in low blood pressure, low energy levels, low blood sugar, and electrolyte imbalances.

Conn's syndrome: an adrenal disorder that causes overproduction of the hormone aldosterone, resulting in excess thirst, excess urination, low potassium levels, muscle weakness, high blood pressure, and over-alkaline blood.

Cretinism: a thyroid disorder in infancy and childhood caused by an inadequately developed thyroid gland, characterized by stunted physical and mental growth.

Cushing's disease: a disease characterized by excessive production of cortisol from the adrenal cortex, resulting in fatty deposits in various locations of the body, weight gain, puffy appearance, chronic fatigue, impotence, a decline in mental ability, and muscle atrophy, among other symptoms.

Diabetes insipidus: a pituitary disorder involving deficient ADH levels, unrelated to diabetes mellitus, that causes very diluted urine; extreme thirst and frequent urination result.

Diabetes mellitus: a pancreatic disorder characterized by chronic hyperglycemia, accompanied by conditions such as peripheral neuropathy, retinopathy, renal impairment, and poor circulation; also called sugar diabetes; classified as type 1 (insulin-dependent) and type 2 (noninsulin-dependent).

Dwarfism: a pituitary disorder caused by a deficiency of growth hormone, characterized by an unusually short stature.

Exophthalmos: abnormal protrusion of the eyeball, sometimes caused by thyroid problems.

Gigantism: a pituitary disorder caused by an excess of growth hormone during childhood, characterized by excessively long bones.

Goiter: a thyroid disorder in which the gland becomes enlarged.

Graves' disease: an autoimmune disorder; the most common cause of hyperthyroidism, which causes bulging eyeballs and an enlarged thyroid (at least double the normal size).

Hashimoto's disease: a nonbacterial inflammation of the thyroid gland, resulting in destruction of the gland and hypothyroidism.

Hyperglycemia: a condition in which the blood sugar level is abnormally high; often characteristic of diabetes mellitus.

Hyperparathyroidism: a disorder in which too much parathyroid hormone is produced, resulting in too much calcium in the blood; causes increased metabolism, high blood pressure, rapid heart rate, and related symptoms.

Hypoglycemia: a deficiency in blood sugar level; can be caused by a diabetic injecting too much insulin or the presence of too little glucose.

Hypoparathyroidism: a disorder in which too little parathyroid hormone is produced, resulting in low blood calcium levels; causes muscle spasms, decreased metabolism, lethargy, sensitivity to cold, and menstrual problems.

Insulin shock: a sudden drop in blood sugar levels resulting from too much insulin being administered that can result in mental impairment, convulsions, and ultimately death if blood sugar is not raised quickly; associated with type 1 diabetes.

Myxedema: a syndrome associated with hypothyroidism; symptoms include edema, weight gain, a slowing of the heart rate, low body temperature, and mental dullness.

Osteitis fibrosa cystica: a parathyroid disorder; a brittleness of the bones caused by an excessive loss of calcium caused by an overactive parathyroid gland.

Seasonal affective disorder (SAD): a pineal disorder, characterized by depressions that occur at the same time every year, usually during winter; symptoms include weight gain, decrease in energy, excessive sleeping, anxiety, and irritability.

Tips for Passing

Try this exercise, called the Cross-Crawl. Standing up, lift your left knee and slap it with your right hand. Then lift your right knee and slap it with your left hand. This activates both sides of your brain and encourages the integration of creative and logical information. Repeat this activity for a minute or so. It's like turning on a light in your brain!

Practice Questions

1. Hormones are composed primarily of
   a. Proteins and steroids
   b. Proteins and sugars
   c. Calcium and magnesium
   d. Potassium and iodine

2. The fight-or-flight response is controlled by the
   a. Pituitary gland
   b. Thyroid gland
   c. Pineal gland
   d. Adrenal glands

3. _____ regulates reproduction in females.
   a. Insulin
   b. Estrogen
   c. Testosterone
   d. Melanin

4. Sex cells are also called
   a. Gonads
   b. Testes
   c. Gametes
   d. Ovaries

5. Insulin is secreted by
   a. The pituitary gland
   b. Lipids
   c. The pancreas
   d. The liver

6. HGH is the acronym for
   a. Human growth hemoglobin
   b. Human gamete hormone
   c. Human growth hormone
   d. Half-growth hormone

7. The general adaptation syndrome is also known as the
   a. Human growth rate
   b. Metabolic response
   c. Stress response
   d. Circadian cycle

Affirmation

I give myself permission to pass this test.

8. The female gonads are the
   a. Ovaries
   b. Testes
   c. Eggs
   d. Uterus

9. The body's metabolism is controlled by the
   a. Hypothalamus
   b. Amygdala
   c. Thyroid
   d. The pituitary

10. If a person is thirsty all the time and has to urinate frequently during the night, that person may have _____.
   a. An infected bladder
   b. Diabetes insipidus
   c. Diabetes mellitus
   d. An enlarged prostate

CHAPTER 14

The Cardiovascular System

Education is for improving the lives of others and for leaving your community and your world better than you found it.

—MARIAN WRIGHT EDELMAN

HIGHLIGHTS

The study of the heart and the circulatory system and its diseases and disorders is known as **cardiology.** The structures of the cardiovascular system include the blood, the heart, and a number of vessels for transporting the blood. The function of the cardiovascular system is to transport the blood throughout the body; the heart acts as the pump.

Blood functions to transport gases, nutrients, and hormones throughout the body tissues; remove waste products from the tissues; regulate the body's **pH** (the acidity or alkalinity); regulate the amounts of fluid present in the tissues; assist in regulating body temperature; and protect against **pathogens.**

Blood is composed of approximately 55% **plasma,** the liquid part of unclotted blood. Plasma is composed of water (90%), with a small amount of proteins (8%) and a smaller amount of salts and acids (2%). The proteins serve different purposes. **Albumins** regulate the blood pressure by functioning like a sponge to keep water in the vascular compartment to maintain plasma volume. **Globulins** help fight infection and transport a variety of substances. **Fibrinogens** cause the blood to clot. Approximately 40% to 50% of the blood consist of **erythrocytes,** or **red blood cells.** The remaining small percentage consists of **leukocytes,** or **white blood cells,** which are the body's main line of defense against infection or illness, and **thrombocytes,** which are cell fragments that contribute to blood clotting.

Coagulation is the process of blood clotting. The blood vessel contracts in response to a local injury; a **platelet plug** (platelets that stick together) forms, and then a clot. The **blood clot,** also referred to as a **thrombus,** is composed of the platelet plugs and binds with blood cells and the walls of the blood vessel. If the clot breaks free and moves through the vessel, it is termed an **embolism. Prothrombin,** which converts to **thrombin,** and **fibrinogen,** which converts to **fibrin,** are proteins known as **clotting factors,** of which there are 11. People who lack any of the clotting factors have a condition called **hemophilia,** which is a tendency to bleed freely.

There are eight different blood types. Their classification depends on the presence or absence of **ABO antigens,** proteins bound to cells that produce specific immune responses in the body and react with the products of that response. The eight blood types are A positive, A negative, B positive, B negative, AB positive, AB negative, O positive, and O negative. O negative blood has no antigens; AB negative contains all existing antigens. **Rh (Rhesus) factor** is a protein that most people have on the surface of their red blood cells. If the Rh factor is present, the person is said to be Rh-positive; without it, the person is Rh-negative. Women who are Rh-negative must take precautions during pregnancy. The majority of babies are born Rh-positive; problems could occur if the baby's blood and the mother's blood become mixed during childbirth, as is likely to happen. In that case, the mother's immune system will start to produce antibodies against Rh-positive blood, creating potential problems for any subsequent pregnancies. This can be avoided by an injection of Rh immunoglobin for the mother.

The **heart** (Fig. 14.1) is a four-chambered pump that contains a number of valves (flaps) that open and close during the delivery of blood. The heart has right and left

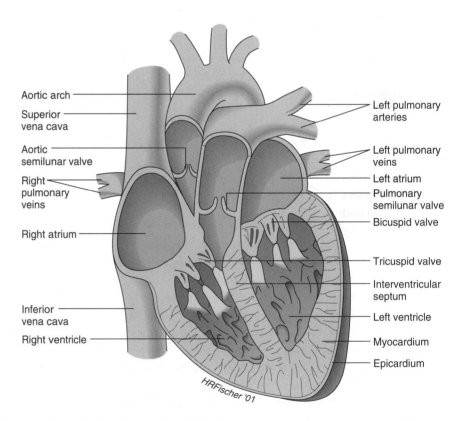

FIGURE 14.1
The major structures of the heart. (Reprinted with permission from Ashton J, Cassel D. Review for Therapeutic Massage and Bodywork Certification. Baltimore: Lippincott Williams & Wilkins, 2002:66.)

ventricles, the muscular chambers that pump blood into pulmonary (right) and systemic (left) circulation; these are separated by a partition called the **interventricular septum.** The two other chambers of the heart, the right and left **atria,** are separated by a partition known as the **interatrial septum.** The right atrium pumps blood into the right ventricle to be sent into pulmonary circulation; the left atrium receives blood returning from the pulmonary veins. The **bicuspid valve,** or **mitral valve,** divides the left atrium from the left ventricle. The bicuspid valve opens to allow blood flow into the left ventricle whenever the left ventricle is relaxed. The **tricuspid** valve divides the right atrium from the right ventricle. The bicuspid and tricuspid valves are both referred to as **atrioventricular (AV) valves.** When the ventricles contract, the AV valves close, preventing the blood from flowing backwards. Instead, the pressure pushes blood out the arteries. The semilunar valves are valves that separate the ventricles from the blood vessels that are attached to them. The **aortic semilunar valve** separates the left ventricle from the aorta; the **pulmonary semilunar valve** separates the right ventricle from the pulmonary trunk. When the ventricles relax, the semilunar valves close to prevent blood in the arteries from flowing backward into the ventricles.

Vessels are the **arteries, arterioles, capillaries, venules,** and **veins** that transport blood. The **great vessels** are the five vessels that are located superior to the aortic arch, the curved part between the ascending and descending parts of the aorta: the carotid artery, the subclavian artery, the brachiocephalic artery, and the right and left brachiocephalic veins. The **aorta** is the largest artery in the body, originating at the heart. The **superior vena cava** is the major vein draining the thorax and the head, ending at the right atrium. The **inferior vena cava** is a large venous trunk draining the lower extremities and the abdomino-pelvic region. The **pulmonary veins** (right and left, superior and inferior) are the only veins that carry oxygenated blood from the lungs to the left atrium. Blood circulates away from the heart through the arteries and capillaries, and back through the veins to return to the heart. The major arteries and veins are shown in Figure 14.2.

Heart sounds are the sounds produced by the closing of the cardiac valves as the heart pumps. **Cardiac output** is a measurement of the volume of blood ejected from the heart (usually the left ventricle) per minute. The **cardiac cycle** is the complete sequence of events from the time one event in the heart occurs until the instant when the same event occurs again. **Systole** is the contraction phase of the cardiac cycle, and **diastole** is the interval between contractions. **Atrial systole** is a contraction of the atrium. **Blood pressure** is the force that circulating blood exerts on the artery walls. The **sinoatrial (SA) node** is called the pacemaker of the heart because it is the impulse-generating tissue that normally dictates heart rate. The SA node is located in the right atrium. The **atrioventricular (AV) node** conducts electrical impulses between the atria and the ventricles. The **atrioventricular bundle** is a bundle of cardiac muscle fibers at the place where the trunk splits into left and right sections. The **heart rate,** or **pulse,** refers to the number of beats per minute. It varies according to whether a person is at rest or in motion and according to a person's age, sex, size, and general health. Heart rate is also affected by stress, nutritional state, and medications.

WHAT YOU NEED TO KNOW

Aorta: the largest artery in the body; it originates at the heart and branches into the extremities, the neck, and all the major organs; supplies oxygenated blood throughout the body.

Aortic valve: a heart valve that divides the left ventricle from the aorta.

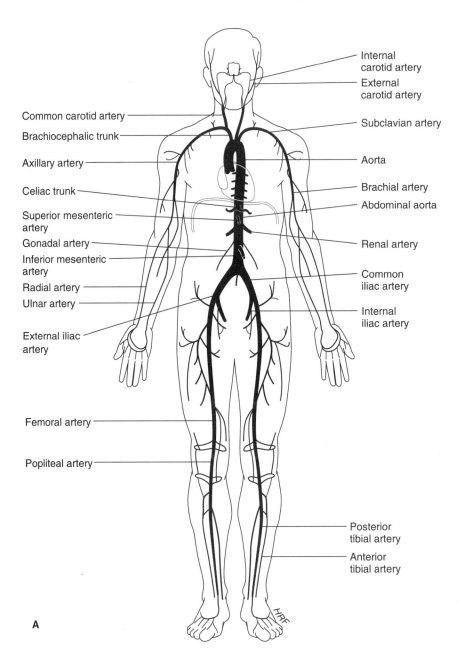

FIGURE 14.2
The body's vessels. **A** The arteries.

Artery: a vessel that carries blood away from the heart.

Atrioventricular (AV) node: a structure located between the atria and the
ventricles that conducts electrical impulses from the atria to the ventricles.

Atrium: one of the two upper (receiving) chambers of the heart.

Baroreceptor: a pressure receptor on the inside walls of some arteries that is
sensitive to stretching of the walls occurring from an increase in pressure.

Bicuspid valve: the heart valve that divides the left atrium from the left ventricle. It
has two flaps, hence its name; also known as the mitral valve.

Bundle branch: a group of specialized cells that rapidly conduct electrical impulses
down into the ventricles.

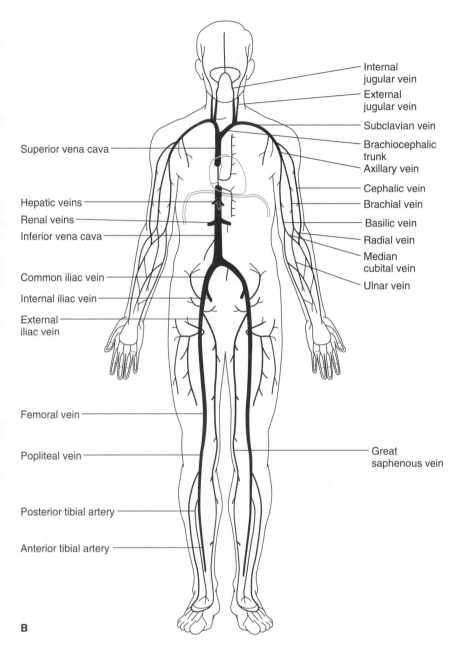

Internal
jugular vein

External
jugular vein

Subclavian vein

Brachiocephalic
trunk

Axillary vein

Cephalic vein

Brachial vein

Basilic vein

Radial vein

Median
cubital vein

Ulnar vein

Great
saphenous vein

Superior vena cava

Hepatic veins

Renal veins

Inferior vena cava

Common iliac vein

Internal iliac vein

External
iliac vein

Femoral vein

Popliteal vein

Posterior tibial artery

Anterior tibial artery

B

FIGURE 14.2 *(continued)*
B The veins. (Reprinted with permission from Ashton J, Cassel D.Review for Therapeutic Massage and Bodywork Certification. Baltimore: Lippincott Williams & Wilkins, 2002:69.)

Capillary: the smallest blood vessel that contains oxygenated blood.

Cardiac cycle: the complete round of circulation from the time one event in the heart occurs until the instant when the same event occurs again.

Cardiac output: a measurement of the volume of blood ejected from the heart per minute. **Cardioinhibitory:** referring to a slowing of the heart rate.

Cardiopulmonary resuscitation (CPR): the A-B-C procedure to artificially return the heartbeat to normal: Establish an *airway*, provide ventilation to restart *breathing*, and perform chest *compressions* to reestablish circulation.

Conduction pathway: cells that are specialized to rapidly spread the electrical signal through the myocardium.

Coronary arteries: the arteries that supply the heart with oxygenated blood.

Coronary sinus: an outlet that drains the five coronary veins into the right atrium.

Diastole: the time it takes in between ventricular contractions for ventricular filling to occur; the phase during which the heart muscle relaxes.

Endocardium: the innermost of the three layers of the heart wall.

Epicardium: the outermost of the three layers of the heart wall.

Heart rate: the number of beats per minute.

Hepatic portal system: a venous system draining the intestines that leads to a second set of capillaries in the liver. From there, blood enters the hepatic portal vein and ultimately the inferior vena cava.

Lumen: the cavity in a blood vessel through which blood flows.

Myocardium: the middle of the three layers forming the wall of the heart; the muscular wall of the heart.

pH scale: the concentration of hydrogen ions, used as a scale to denote acidity or alkalinity.

Pulmonary circulation: the circulation of blood through the lungs.

Pulmonary valve: a valve that divides the right ventricle and the pulmonary artery.

Pulmonary veins: veins that return oxygenated blood from the lungs to the left atrium.

Purkinje fibers: a type of fiber that stimulates the contraction of the myocardium.

Sinoatrial (SA) node: the pacemaker tissue of the heart; an impulse-generating tissue.

Stroke volume: the amount of blood that is pumped out of one ventricle as a result of one contraction of the cardiac muscle.

Vasoconstrictor: a nerve or substance that causes a blood vessel to constrict.

Vasodilator: a nerve or substance that causes a blood vessel to dilate.

Vein: a vessel that carries blood toward the heart.

Ventricle: the chamber of the heart responsible for pumping the blood.

Venule: a tiny vessel that collectively forms veins.

PATHOLOGY OF THE CARDIOVASCULAR SYSTEM

Many factors are involved in the pathology of the cardiovascular system, with cigarette smoking and diet being two of the major contributors to heart disease and/or heart attack and stroke. According to the American Heart Association, more than one million Americans experience a heart attack every year. Heart disease is the leading cause of death in American women. High blood pressure is a risk factor, and so are sedentary lifestyle, high cholesterol levels, stress, excessive alcohol or drug abuse, obesity, and family predisposition. Other conditions, such as diabetes, can also raise the risk of cardiovascular disease.

Anaphylactic shock: a life-threatening allergic reaction resulting in difficulty breathing and low blood pressure.

Anemia: a deficiency of red blood cells that results in too little oxygen reaching tissues and organs.

Aneurysm: a blood-filled, pulsing sac formed by the dilation of the wall of an artery or vein.

Angina: chest pain resulting from inadequate oxygen reaching the heart muscle, characterized by a "squeezing" feeling in the middle chest; usually caused by atherosclerosis.

Anoxia: a total lack of oxygen in the tissues.

Aplastic anemia: a condition resulting from the bone marrow producing too few red and white blood cells; too little oxygen reaches the organs and tissues; the usual causes are drugs, radiation, and/or cancer.

Arrhythmia: an irregular heartbeat.

Arteriosclerosis: a general term for hardening or calcification of the arteries.

Atherosclerosis: a progressive narrowing and hardening of the walls of the arteries caused by fatty deposits that build on the inner walls of the arteries and interfere with blood flow.

Bone marrow suppression: a decrease in red and white blood cells and platelets, leading to anemia, increased risk for infections, and excess bleeding.

Bradycardia: an unusual slowness of the heartbeat.

Cardiac arrest: a complete shutdown of the heart's pumping action, possibly caused by a heart attack, respiratory arrest, electrical shock, extreme cold, blood loss, drug overdose, or severe allergic reaction.

Cardiogenic shock: inadequate oxygen delivery to the tissues caused by heart failure, causing depression of all body functions.

Coarctation of the aorta: a birth defect that results in the aorta being too narrow for sufficient blood transport.

Congestive heart failure: an insufficient pumping action of the heart that leads to an accumulation of fluid in the lungs, causing shortness of breath and swelling of the lower extremities.

Coronary artery disease: a narrowing of the arteries that prevents adequate blood flow to the heart, ultimately resulting in a heart attack.

Cyanosis: a blue tint to the skin, nails, or mucus membranes resulting from a lack of oxygen in the arterial blood.

Deep vein thrombosis: blood clots in the veins of the inner thigh or leg that have the potential to break off and go to the lungs, causing respiratory distress or failure.

Edema: swelling caused by abnormal accumulation of fluid in the extracellular space.

Embolus: a blood clot that forms in the vessel in one part of the body and travels to another part.

Gangrene: tissue death from a lack of oxygen or nutrients, resulting in bacterial infection and putrefaction.

Heart block: the delay or complete block of electrical impulses in the heart.

Hemolytic anemia: an anemia resulting from red cells that survive an abnormally short time.

Hemophilia: a genetic condition characterized by the absence of clotting factors in the blood; those with hemophilia are often termed "free bleeders."

Hemorrhagic anemia: anemia resulting from a loss of blood.

Hemorrhoid: a painful swelling varicosity around the opening of the anus.

Hypertension: persistently high blood pressure.

Hypotension: abnormally low blood pressure.

Hypovolemic shock: abnormally low levels of plasma in the blood, resulting in the inability to maintain proper blood pressure and tissue function, and profound physical depression of the entire body.

Hypoxia: a decrease of oxygen to an area even though there may be adequate blood flow.

Leukemia: a malignancy of the blood-forming tissue, causing a seriously abnormal increase of leukocytes (white blood cells) in the tissue.

Mitral valve prolapse: a floppy bicuspid valve that is working incorrectly; usually causes no symptoms.

Myocardial infarction: an irreversible injury to the heart muscle; commonly known as a heart attack.

Myocardial ischemia: abnormal heart function caused by a lack of sufficient oxygen to the heart muscle; may lead to electrical arrhythmias, mechanical dysfunction of the heart, angina, or myocardial infarction.

Murmur: an abnormal heart sound most often caused by heart valves not functioning correctly.

Necrosis: cell death caused by disease or injury; may progress to include tissue and organ damage.

Nutritional anemia: anemia caused by a dietary deficiency of iron, folic acid, vitamins, or proteins necessary to build red blood cells.

Patent ductus arteriosus: a birth defect causing the normal channel between the aorta and the pulmonary artery to fail to close.

Pericarditis: an inflammation of the pericardium.

Pernicious anemia: an anemia caused by an insufficient number of red blood cells caused by the lack of vitamin B12 in the body.

Phlebitis: the inflammation of a vein.

Raynaud's disease: blood vessel spasms in the fingers and toe, resulting in pallor (discoloration); indicative of a lack of circulation.

Septal defect: a birth defect involving a hole in the wall between the upper chambers of the heart.

Septicemia: the presence of bacteria in the blood.

Septic shock: a frequently fatal type of shock that often accompanies burns or traumatic abdominal wounds resulting from endotoxins (toxin-like cells that bind to bacteria) released by the infecting bacteria.

Sickle-cell anemia: a type of blood disease common in African Americans and others who originate in areas where malaria is common; blood cells change from their normal disc-like shape into a sickle shape and can become damaged or trapped in the capillaries, resulting in insufficient oxygen for normal tissue and organ function.

Tachycardia: an excessively rapid heartbeat, usually classified as more than 100 beats per minute.

Tetralogy of Fallot: a congenital birth defect in which the aorta is on the wrong side (right instead of left); the most serious of several heart conditions occurring together and resulting in a "blue baby" from lack of oxygen. Emergency surgery must be performed for the baby's survival.

Thrombophlebitis: an inflammation of a vein with the potential for blood clotting.

Varicose vein: an abnormal swelling of the veins of the legs.

Tips for Passing

Read very carefully and pay special attention to questions that contain negative wording, such as "least" or "not." Be very alert for double or triple negatives that can entirely change the meaning of the question.

Practice Questions

1. The body's main line of defense against infection or illness are the
   a. Erythrocytes
   b. Leukocytes
   c. Fibrinogens
   d. Hematites

2. There are _____ different blood types.
   a. 8
   b. 6
   c. 9
   d. 5

3. The largest artery in the body is the
   a. Jugular vein
   b. Subclavian
   c. Aorta
   d. Thrombus

4. The smallest blood vessels that carry oxygenated blood are the
   a. Varicose veins
   b. Brachial arteries
   c. Capillaries
   d. Coronary arteries

5. A complete shutdown of the heart is a
   a. Cardiac arrest
   b. Cardiovascular episode
   c. Mitral valve prolapse
   d. CVA

6. A genetic condition that results in a lack of clotting factors in the blood is
   a. Hypochondria
   b. Sickle-cell anemia
   c. Hyperion anemia
   d. Hemophilia

7. Hypertension is the condition of
   a. Attention deficit disorder
   b. Low blood pressure
   c. Heart murmur
   d. High blood pressure

8. An excessively rapid heartbeat is known as
   a. Nascardia
   b. Brachycardia

Affirmation

I enjoy my life while completing my goals.

    c. Angina

    d. Tachycardia

9. A progressive narrowing and hardening of the arteries caused by age, high cholesterol levels, smoking, and/or other factors is called

    a. Cerebrovascular accident

    b. Cyanosis

    c. Atherosclerosis

    d. Scleroderma

10. An inflammation of the veins is called

    a. Varicose veins

    b. Necrosis

    c. Phlebitis

    d. Bursitis

CHAPTER 15

The Lymphatic and Immune Systems

Education is not the filling of a pail, but the lighting of a fire.
— W.B. YEATS

HIGHLIGHTS

The structures of the lymphatic system consist of the fluid called **lymph,** the **lymphatic vessels** that transport it, and several different structures that house lymphatic tissue. Lymph originates from interstitial fluid and contains a lot of **lymphocytes,** the white cells of the blood that fight infection. The lymphatic system is a specialized, pumpless, vascular system that performs three basic functions: drains excess **interstitial fluid** through the lymphatic vessels, transports lipids and vitamins, and protects the body through immune responses.

Located throughout the body along the lymphatic vessels are approximately 600 bean-sized organs called **lymph nodes.** The major nodes are named according to location:

- Axillary (under the arm)
- Cubital (at the elbow)
- Deep cervical (deep in the neck)
- Superficial cervical (superficial in the neck)
- Deep inguinal (deep in the groin)
- Superficial inguinal (superficial in the groin)
- Facial (at the medial angle of the eye)
- Femoral (at the femur)
- Hypogastric (at the lower abdomen)
- Mediastinal (behind the sternum)

- Mesenteric (in and around abdominal membranes)
- Occipital (at the back of the head)
- Para-aortic (below the diaphragm)
- Parotid (in front of the ear)
- Popliteal (on the back of the knee)
- Subclavicular (under the clavicle)
- Submandibular (under the mandible)
- Supratrochlear (above the eye)
- Tibial (at the tibia)

The lymphatic system's major components are shown in Figure 15.1. Because the lymphatic system is complex, make it a point to study an anatomy textbook for a more detailed look at the system.

Lymph is also referred to as interstitial fluid or plasma; excess fluid migrates from the spaces between the cells into the **lymphatic capillaries** and from there into the lymphatic vessels because of **osmotic pressure.** The movement of lymph is facilitated by the skeletal muscles. If the lymph vessels did not act to remove the excess fluid, **edema** (also called **lymphedema**) would result.

The organs of the lymphatic system are divided into two classes, primary and secondary. The **primary lymphatic organs** provide a growing environment for stem cell division into **B cells** and **T cells,** the lymphocytes that carry out the body's immune response. The primary organs are the red bone marrow and the thymus gland. After the B and T cells have been manufactured in the **red bone marrow,** the T cells move to the **thymus gland** where they mature; B cells remain in the bone marrow to mature. The **secondary lymphatic organs** are the lymph nodes, the **lymphatic nodules** (tissue, not an actual organ), and the **spleen,** the largest lymphatic organ in the body.

The **left lymphatic duct,** also called the **thoracic duct,** is the major efferent duct into which most of the peripheral lymph nodes drain. The thoracic duct is approximately 16 inches long. It is the main collecting duct of the lymphatic system. It drains lymph from the left side of the head, neck, and thorax, the left upper extremity, and the entire body below the ribs. It empties lymph into the left subclavian veins, which are located underneath our collarbones. The **right lymphatic duct** is on the right side of the lower neck and empties into the **brachiocephalic vein.** The **lymphatic plexus** is a network of lymphatic capillaries that opens into one or more of the larger lymphatic vessels. There are three lymphatic plexuses: the mammary plexus, positioned around the internal thoracic veins; the palmar plexus, positioned around the venous arch where the radial and ulnar veins arise; and the plantar plexus, positioned in the deep plantar surface of the foot.

The most important function of the lymphatic system is its interaction with the immune system in protecting the body from invaders through **immune responses.** The body's ability to ward off illness is called **resistance;** the lack of resistance is known as **susceptibility.** Resistance can also be referred to as **immunity.** There are two different types of immunity: nonspecific and specific. **Nonspecific immunity,** often called **general immunity,** consists of the body's natural defenses that do not differentiate between potential invaders. The components of nonspecific immunity include our normal excretions, such as mucus, sweat, and earwax; the **inflammatory response;** reflex responses, such as coughing, sneezing, and fever; flora, the bacteria that live in the integumentary and digestive systems and serve to prevent harmful bacteria from damaging the body; and natural body defenses, such as **phagocytes** and **interferon.**

Specific immunity is the body's resistance as a result of exposure to a specific **antigen** from a foreign cell. A good example is naturally occurring immunity because of exposure to a foreign antigen, such as a child contracting measles; immunity from

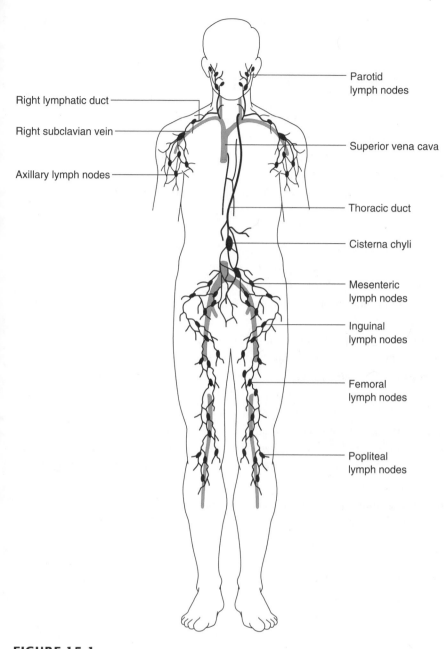

FIGURE 15.1
The body's major lymph nodes and lymph vessels. (Reprinted with permission from Ashton J, Cassel D. Review for Therapeutic Massage and Bodywork Certification. Baltimore: Lippincott Williams & Wilkins, 2002:72.)

that disease in the future will develop in that child. Specific immunity also refers to **acquired immunity,** such as immunity by means of a **vaccination.** There are four classifications of acquired immunity:

1. **Active naturally acquired immunity:** immunity acquired naturally by exposure to a foreign antigen, such as that for the chicken pox virus.
2. **Passive naturally acquired immunity:** immunity acquired through the placenta or through the breast milk of a nursing mother.
3. **Active artificially acquired immunity:** immunity acquired as the result of a vaccine (gammaglobulin shot).

4. **Passive artificially acquired immunity:** immunity from antibodies taken from one person and given to another.

WHAT YOU NEED TO KNOW

Antibody: a protein molecule produced by B cells; antibodies are the primary immune system defense.

Antigen: a substance that can cause a specific immune response and then reacts with the products of the response.

Axillary lymph nodes: nodes around the axillary (armpit) area that receive lymph drainage from the upper arm and the scapular and pectoral regions; they drain into the subclavian trunk.

B cell: a type of lymphocyte that specializes in producing antibodies.

Cisterna chyli: a sac on the inferior portion of the thoracic duct that holds chyle, a milky yellow fluid that drains from the intestines.

Complement system: an immune defense system of plasma proteins that destroy microbes.

Cytokine: a protein released by cells that affects cell-to-cell communication and interactions; cytokines have similar actions to hormones.

Gamma globulin: one of several types of antibodies; a protein derived from blood that has been infected with a pathogen; antibodies are created, isolated, and injected into the human to cause short-term immunity.

Inguinal lymph node: one of several small nodes deep to the tensor fascia lata that receive lymph drainage from the deep structures of the lower limbs.

Interferon: a natural cytokine secreted by the body to keep viruses from infecting cells and replicating.

Lacteal: one of the lymphatic vessels that transports a milky fluid (chyle) through the small intestine and the mesenteric glands to the thoracic ducts.

Lumbar lymph node: one of a chain of lymph nodes located around the inferior vena cava.

Lymph capillary: the beginning of a lymphatic vessel.

Lymph duct: a tube that allows the passage of lymph from one place to another.

Lymph node: a bean-sized organ located throughout the body; lymph nodes filter out antigens and are the site of antigen presentation and immune activation.

Mandibular lymph node: a facial lymph node that is located at the point where the facial artery crosses the mandible.

Memory cell: a cell that remains after the body mounts an immune response to an antigen and is capable of an immediate response to the reappearance of the same antigen. Memory cells include certain subsets of T cells and some B cells.

Mesenteric lymph node: a node located in and around the abdominal membranes.

Palatine tonsils: a large oval-shaped mass of lymphatic tissue located in the wall of the pharynx at the back of the throat; the structure commonly referred to as the tonsils.

Phagocyte: cells capable of "swallowing up" other cells (harmful ones) and even digesting them.

Pharyngeal tonsils: a group of small lymphatic nodules located on the back and roof of the nasopharynx; those that grow too large (and are often surgically removed in children) are called adenoids.

Popliteal lymph nodes: two groups of nodes located around the back of the knee that drain the skin of the posterior leg, deep structures of the leg, and side of the foot.

T cell: a type of cell derived from the thymus that helps coordinate immune system functions through the secretion of hormones.

T-cytotoxic cells: specialized T cells that destroy infected or other diseased cells, including cancer cells; the most significant component of the cellular immune response.

T-helper cell: a type of T cell that regulates the immune response.

Thoracic duct: the major efferent lymph duct into which most lymph nodes drain; also called the left lymphatic duct.

Tonsils: lymphatic tissues covered by a membrane and located on either side of the throat.

PATHOLOGY OF THE LYMPHATIC AND IMMUNE SYSTEMS

The pathology of the lymphatic and immune systems consists of diseases that are caused by some type of dysfunction in the immune system. Remember, though, that the lymphatic and immune systems are the body's defense against infectious agents and abnormal cells. Failure of the immune system includes some genetic conditions. There are also autoimmune disorders in which the immune system fails or even attacks itself, leaving the body vulnerable to multiple symptoms and chronic illness that can lead to death.

As a massage therapist, you need to be aware of contraindications related to the lymphatic system. It is impossible to give a massage without affecting lymphatic structures and flow. Any cancer involving the lymphatic system is a classic contraindication to massage. Don't forget that the lymphatic system is the body's immune defense, so you want to avoid doing anything to compromise that critical function.

Abscess: a localized collection of pus caused by an infection.

Acute lymphoblastic leukemia: the most common type of childhood leukemia; a rapidly growing cancer of the blood causing an abnormal increase in white blood cells. (A chronic instead of acute form is slow-growing.)

Acute myeloblastic leukemia: a type of cancer of the blood that usually affects adults; it affects the immature blood cells in the bone marrow. (A chronic instead of acute form is slow-growing.)

Adenitis: an inflammation of a gland.

AIDS (acquired immunodeficiency syndrome): a disease caused by infection from the human immunodeficiency virus (HIV), which attacks the immune system and causes it to eventually fail.

Allergy: a hypersensitivity to a particular allergen, resulting in harmful reactions on subsequent exposures.

Burkitt's lymphoma: a type of non-Hodgkin's lymphoma that causes a fast-growing tumor in the abdomen of children; thought to be associated with Epstein–Barr virus.

Chronic fatigue syndrome: an illness of unknown origin, characterized by extreme fatigue, swelling of the lymph nodes, muscle aches, and general weakness; also thought to be associated with Epstein–Barr virus.

Edema: swelling caused by abnormal amounts of fluid in the intercellular tissue spaces of the body.

Elephantiasis: a rare disorder of the lymphatic system caused by parasitic worms that are transmitted by mosquitos, in which inflammation and blockage of the lymphatic vessels causes extreme edema formation and enlargement of the affected area, most commonly a limb or parts of the head and torso.

Epstein–Barr virus: a herpes virus that causes infectious mononucleosis; also thought to be associated with Burkitt's lymphoma and chronic fatigue syndrome.

Fever: a physiological response to infection and or inflammation, wherein the body's temperature rises above normal.

Hodgkin's disease: a malignant illness that begins with infection in one lymph node and progressively spreads throughout the lymphatic system, into the spleen, liver, and eventually the bone marrow.

Leukemia: an acute or chronic cancerous disease characterized by a seriously abnormal increase of leukocytes (white blood cells) in the tissue; there may or may not be an increase in the number of leukocytes in the circulating blood; cause unknown.

Lymphedema: fluid accumulation under the skin caused by obstructed lymph, characterized by a swelling of the tissues, especially in the extremities.

Lymphoma: a malignant tumor occurring in the lymphatic system.

Mononucleosis: an acute infection of the lymphatic tissue caused by the Epstein–Barr virus; characterized by fever and swollen lymph nodes and an abnormal increase of mononuclear leukocytes or monocytes in the bloodstream; also called kissing disease because the virus is transmitted in saliva.

Rejection: nonacceptance of transplanted or grafted tissue in the body.

Splenomegaly: an enlargement of the spleen.

Systemic lupus erythematosus: a chronic, inflammatory, immune complex disorder, resulting from an immune system malfunction that causes antibodies and antibody–antigen complexes to be produced to the victim's own tissues; severe inflammations and organ damage often occur. Usually referred to as lupus.

 Tips for Passing

Whether or not your particular massage school covered lymphatic massage, schedule a massage with a specialist in lymphatic drainage massage, and ask her to explain what she is doing. There is nothing like a hands-on experience to help get something to stick in the brain. Although there are several different techniques of lymphatic massage, they are all based on the same anatomical and physiological facts. If you tell the therapist you are studying for the examination, she will probably be very helpful to you. Besides, the lymph drainage will do you good.

Practice Questions

1. The function of lymph is to
   a. Drain excess interstitial fluid
   b. Transport lipids and vitamins
   c. Protect the body through immune response
   d. All of the above

2. Lymphocytes are also known as
   a. B cells and C cells
   b. L cells and C cells
   c. B cells and T cells
   d. D cells and C cells

3. Immunity acquired as the result of a vaccine is called
   a. Passive naturally acquired immunity
   b. Active naturally acquired immunity
   c. Passive artificially required immunity
   d. Active artificially acquired immunity

4. Proteins that regulate many cell functions are called
   a. Cytokines
   b. Leukocytes
   c. Lymphocytes
   d. Gamma cells

5. The popliteal lymph nodes are located
   a. Under the clavicle
   b. Next to the maxilla
   c. Behind the knee
   d. At the greater trochanter

6. A malignant illness that begins with the infection of one lymph node is
   a. Alzheimer's disease
   b. Fibromyalgia
   c. Hodgkin's disease
   d. Huntington's disease

7. The lymphatic tissues that are covered by a membrane and located on either side of the throat are the
   a. Pharynx
   b. Larynx
   c. Tonsils
   d. Hyoid

8. Fluid accumulation resulting in swelling is known as
   a. Lymphago
   b. Lumbago
   c. Lymphedema
   d. Sacofluidesis

9. An enlargement of the spleen is called
   a. Splenomegaly
   b. Splenomyoly
   c. Splenocitis
   d. Splenojumbo

10. AIDS is the acronym for
   a. Active immunodeficiency syndrome
   b. Acquired immunodeficiency syndrome
   c. Antibody immunodeficiency syndrome
   d. Antigen immunodeficiency syndrome

CHAPTER 16

The Respiratory System

Learning is not attained by chance, it must be sought for with ardor and attended to with diligence.

—ABIGAIL ADAMS

HIGHLIGHTS

The structures of the respiratory system include the nose, pharynx (throat), larynx (voice box), trachea (windpipe), bronchi, and lungs. The **upper respiratory tract** includes the nose, pharynx, larynx, and associated tissues; the **lower respiratory system** includes the trachea, bronchi, and lungs. The main structures of the respiratory system are illustrated in Figure 16.1.

The **nose** contains the **nostrils (nares)** and the **olfactory cavity.** The term *nares* also refers to the nasal openings in the **nasal cavities** in the back of the mouth, in the area called the **nasopharynx.** The nostrils are lined with **cilia,** fine hairs that serve as filters for the respiratory system. The nose is the **olfactory organ,** located in the superior part of the nasal cavity. It is the organ of smell. The **olfactory nerve** (cranial nerve I) is responsible for nerve impulses to the brain that enable us to recognize different smells. The **nasolacrimal apparatus** causes our eyes to tear when confronted with an acrid smell. The **nasal reflex response** causes us to sneeze whenever our mucous membranes are irritated. The **sinuses** are air-filled cavities in the facial structure. The **turbinates,** or **conchae,** are the bony plates with curving margins on the lateral walls of the nasal cavity. The **meatus** refers to any of the three passages in the nasal cavity formed by the conchae.

The **pharynx** is the throat, the cavity at the back of the mouth. It is shaped like a cone, made of skeletal muscle, and has a mucous membrane lining. The pharynx is a passageway for air, water, and food, and is a resonating chamber for sound. Food

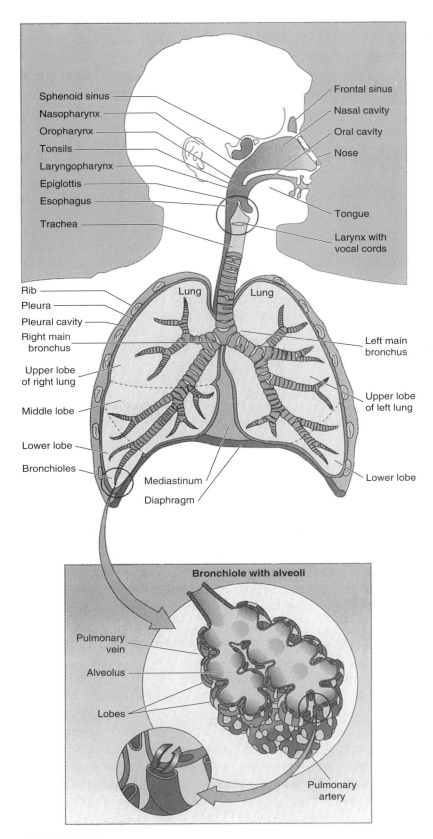

FIGURE 16.1

Components of the respiratory system. (Reprinted with permission from Willis MC. Medical Terminology: The Language of Health Care, 1st ed. Baltimore: Williams & Wilkins, 1996:A18.)

and water move from the pharynx into the **esophagus.** The **tonsils** are located in the pharynx, but they are part of the lymphatic system and not the respiratory system proper.

The **larynx** (voice box) is a passageway from the pharynx to the trachea. The larynx is composed of cartilages that are connected to each other and to other structures of the throat. The **glottis,** which is made up of the **true vocal cords** and the opening between them **(rima glottidis),** is the vocal apparatus. The **epiglottis** is like a lid that closes the glottis while food or liquid is passing through the pharynx. Superior to the true vocal cords, which are a pair of folds in the mucosal lining of the larynx, is a second pair of folds called the **false vocal cords.**

The **trachea** (windpipe) is made of hyaline cartilage and lined with a mucous membrane. It is the passageway between the larynx and the **bronchi.** The bronchi are divided into the **right and left primary bronchi,** which lead into the right and left lungs. On entering the lungs, they are divided further into the **secondary (lobar) bronchi.** They continue to branch into smaller bronchi, the **segmental (tertiary) bronchi.** These in turn branch into still smaller bronchi called **bronchioles,** which in turn have even smaller appendages known as **terminal bronchioles.** The entire bronchial system looks like an upside-down tree and is often referred to as the **bronchial tree.** The bronchi can be constricted or dilated like blood vessels, whether caused by illness or chemical or mechanical intervention; these processes are referred to as **bronchoconstriction** and **bronchodilation.**

The **lungs** are the pair of breathing organs located in the **thoracic cavity,** which is divided in two by the **mediastinum.** Their action is to rid the body of excess carbon dioxide and to bring in fresh oxygen. They take up most of the space in the **thorax.** The lungs are separated from each other by the heart, and each resides in a distinct chamber, so it is possible that trauma or injury affecting one lung may not affect the other. The lungs are divided into **lobes** and are covered by a protective two-layered membrane called the **pleural membrane.** The right lung is divided into three lobes. The left lung is smaller to accommodate the heart and only has two lobes. The outer layer of the pleural membrane, the **parietal pleura,** lines the walls of the thoracic cavity. The inner layer of the pleural membrane, the **visceral pleura,** covers the actual lungs. Between the parietal and visceral pleura is the **pleural space,** also referred to as the **pleural cavity.**

During inhalation, the **diaphragm** contracts and flattens in conjunction with the other muscles of respiration to increase the size of the thoracic cavity and make room for air to be drawn into the lungs. On exhalation, the same muscles relax to release air from the lungs.

The function of the respiratory system is gas exchange within the body, referred to as **respiration.** Respiration occurs in three steps: **pulmonary ventilation** (breathing), the flowing of air in and out of the lungs; **external respiration,** the exchange of gases between the air spaces in the lungs and the blood in the pulmonary capillaries; and **internal respiration,** the exchange of gases between the blood in systemic capillaries and tissue cells.

Inhalation, the act of breathing in, is also referred to as **inspiration.** Normal inhalation is referred to as **quiet inspiration. Deep inspiration** is also referred to as **forced inspiration.** Exhalation, the act of normally breathing out, is also referred to as **quiet expiration.** Labored exhalation is referred to as **forced expiration.** The **respiratory rate** is the number of breaths we take each minute and is normally measured by counting the number of times the chest rises (or falls) per minute. The average adult takes approximately 12 breaths per minute, but it varies based on size, health, whether the person smokes, and so on. **Eupnea** is the term for normal, resting breathing.

The respiratory system enables the body to respond to emotional stimuli as well as foreign objects. **Yawning** is an involuntary inhalation with the mouth open. Although scientifically it is not clearly understood, yawning may be the body's signal for needing more oxygen (to stay awake, for instance) or it may be a stress relief mechanism. **Sighing** is a deep inhalation followed by a short, forceful expiration. Sighing is a stress relief mechanism. One of my instructors used to refer to a sigh as a "brain shower," a moment of giving your brain a rest (sigh right now, if you want to). **Crying, sobbing,** and **laughing** are all functions of the respiratory system and are in fact all caused by convulsive inspirations and/or expirations. Laughing and crying are sometimes indistinguishable from each other.

A **sneeze** is an involuntary expiration through the nose and mouth that occurs by reflex action whenever the mucous membranes of the nose are irritated. A **cough** is an expulsion of air from the lungs through the mouth in order to clear the lungs or passages of mucus, fluid, or foreign substances. A **hiccup** is a spasmodic contraction of the diaphragm followed by a spasmodic closing of the glottis that results in an abnormally sharp sound while breathing in; it is usually caused by an irritation of the afferent nerve endings in the GI tract. **Valsalva's maneuver** is the act, voluntary or involuntary, of forced expiration against the closed glottis during straining, such as straining to defecate or trying to equalize sinus pressure while adjusting to altitude.

The cells in the body continually burn oxygen to fuel **metabolism;** in turn, metabolic reactions produce an excess of carbon dioxide, which must be eliminated quickly from the body. During external respiration, the blood in the **pulmonary capillaries** gains oxygen while releasing **carbon dioxide.** During internal respiration, the blood in the **systemic capillaries** loses oxygen and gains carbon dioxide.

The respiratory system functions in two main portions. The **conducting portion** can be thought of as the **air filter.** The conducting portion is actually a series of cavities and tubes connected to each other, whose purpose is to filter, warm, and moisten the air before conducting it into the lungs; it consists of the nose, pharynx, larynx, trachea, bronchi, bronchioles, and terminal bronchioles. The **respiratory portion** refers to the actual tissues of the lungs where gas exchange takes place: the **respiratory bronchioles, alveolar ducts, alveolar sacs,** and **alveoli.**

The study of the respiratory system has two specialties. **Pulmonology** refers to the study of the lungs, and the diagnosis, treatment, and prevention of lung diseases. **Otorhinolaryngology** refers to the study of the ears, nose, and throat, and the diagnosis, treatment, and prevention of disease in those organs.

WHAT YOU NEED TO KNOW

Alveoli: small sacs in the lungs that fill with air from the alveolar ducts. Singular: alveolus.

Bronchi: the larger air passages in the lungs. Singular: bronchus.

Bronchiole: a tiny branch of the bronchi that connects to the alveoli.

Choana: the outer curved part of the nasal cavities that acts as a filter for dust, to warm and moisten the incoming air.

Diaphragm: a dome-shaped muscle between the thoracic and abdominal cavities; controls regular, relaxed breathing by contracting and relaxing.

Epiglottis: a cartilaginous flap above the glottis that closes while food or liquid is passing through the pharynx.

Exhalation: breathing out.

Expiration: breathing out.

Glottis: the vocal cords and the opening between them.

Inhalation: breathing in.

Inspiration: breathing in; the act of drawing air into the lungs.

Laryngopharynx: the bottom part of the pharynx.

Larynx: the voice box.

Lungs: the main breathing organs in the chest that bring oxygen into the body and expel carbon dioxide.

Nasal cavity: any of the openings in the nasal passages.

Nasopharynx: the part of the pharynx behind the nasal cavity and above the soft palate.

Nostrils: external openings of the nose that provide air passage and secretions from the nose and eyes.

Oropharynx: the part of the throat located at the back of the mouth.

Parietal pleura: the outer layer of the pleural membrane.

Pharynx: the cavity at the back of the mouth that opens to the esophagus and larynx.

Residual volume: the volume of air left in the lungs after a maximum exhalation.

Sinus: an air-filled cavity.

Tidal volume: the volume of air that is inhaled or exhaled during a normal, resting breathing cycle.

Total lung capacity: the volume of air in the lungs after a maximum inhalation.

Visceral pleura: the inner layer of the pleural membrane.

Vital capacity: the volume of gas that can be exhaled from the lungs at maximum inhalation.

PATHOLOGY OF THE RESPIRATORY SYSTEM

As with the cardiovascular system, the common contributor to illnesses of the respiratory system is cigarette smoking. The chemicals in cigarette smoke over time destroy the ciliated epithelial cells in the airways and cause excess mucus production. The tar and nicotine in cigarette smoke are the primary cause of **lung cancer.** Second-hand smoke is a danger to those who don't smoke; studies have shown that children of smokers are more prone to respiratory illnesses than children who have nonsmoking parents. Damage to the respiratory system from cigarette smoking is slow, progressive, and deadly. A healthy respiratory system is continuously cleansed by the filtering action of the mucous membranes and the cilia. The mucus produced by the respiratory tubules traps dirt and disease-causing organisms, which cilia sweep toward the mouth, where it can be eliminated. Smoking greatly impairs this process. With the very first inhalation of smoke, the beating of the cilia slows down; over time, the cilia become paralyzed and eventually disappear altogether. The loss of cilia leads to the development of smoker's cough. Because the cilia can no longer effectively remove mucus, the individual must cough it up. Coughing is usually worse in the morning because mucus accumulates during sleep. Excess mucus accumulates and starts blocking the air passages, making breathing difficult because the body's natural line of defense, the air-filtering system, has been destroyed by cigarette smoke. Lung cancer is one of the most deadly forms of cancer with one of the highest mortality rates. The American

Cancer Society states that only 13% of lung cancer victims will still be alive 5 years after their cancer is diagnosed.

Emphysema is a lung disease in which tissue deterioration results in increased air retention and reduced exchange of gases. The result is difficult breathing and shortness of breath. Emphysema and chronic bronchitis can also result in **chronic obstructive pulmonary disease (COPD),** a progressive disease characterized by shortness of breath, wheezing, and chronic coughing, usually caused by smoking.

Influenza (flu), an acute viral infection involving the respiratory tract as well as the other body systems, is widespread. Children, the elderly, and anyone with a compromised immune system are in more danger of getting the flu than the average healthy adult. Precautions can be taken to prevent the spread of influenza, and staying away from those who have it is the number one recommendation. Influenza is a definite contraindication for massage—for your own safety as well as your client's.

Acute respiratory distress syndrome (ARDS): a number of conditions in which the lungs receive inadequate oxygen; may be caused by a pathological condition or to exposure to smoke, pollution, or toxic chemicals, resulting in shortness of breath.

Apnea: the temporary cessation of breathing (usually occurs during sleep).

Asphyxia: a condition caused by an inadequate intake of oxygen.

Aspiration: the accidental inhalation of foreign matter into the bronchial system.

Asthma: a disease characterized by narrowing of the bronchial tubes, making breathing difficult.

Bradypnea: abnormally slow breathing.

Bronchitis: the inflammation of the bronchi.

Cheyne–Stokes respiration: an irregular breathing pattern consisting of periods of maximum respiration followed by a progressive decrease until apnea results; often seen in comatose or brain-injured patients.

Chronic obstructive pulmonary disease (COPD): a progressive disease characterized by shortness of breath, wheezing, and chronic coughing, usually caused by smoking; usually a combination of chronic bronchitis and emphysema.

Coryza: profuse discharge from the mucous membrane of the nose.

Cystic fibrosis: a common genetic disorder of infants and children in which thick, viscous mucus is produced in the respiratory tract; the exocrine glands do not secrete properly, and a predisposition to bacterial infections exists in the lungs.

Dyspnea: shortness of breath.

Emphysema: a lung disease in which tissue deterioration results in increased air retention and reduced exchange of gases. The result is difficult breathing and shortness of breath; usually caused by smoking.

Epistaxis: a common nosebleed.

Hay fever: a seasonal rhinitis resulting from an allergic reaction to pollen.

Hemoptysis: coughing up blood from the lungs or airways.

Hiccup: an involuntary spastic contraction of the diaphragm.

Hyperventilation: abnormally deep or fast respiration, in which excessive quantities of air are taken in, causing buzzing in the ears, tingling in the extremities, and, sometimes, fainting.

Influenza: an acute viral infection involving the respiratory tract and the other body systems.

Lung cancer: a cancerous growth in the lung tissue.

Pleurisy: an inflammation of the covering around the lungs.

Pneumonia: an inflammation of the lungs caused by a bacterial or viral infection, which causes fever, shortness of breath, and the coughing up of phlegm (mucus and other material produced by the lining of the respiratory tract; also called sputum).

Pneumothorax: a collapsed lung caused by accumulation of air or gas in the space between the lung and chest wall.

Pulmonary edema: the abnormal collection of fluid in the lungs.

Respiratory failure: an inability of the lungs to conduct gas exchange.

Respiratory hypersensitivity: asthma, hay fever, and other conditions caused by an oversensitivity of any part of the respiratory system.

Respiratory insufficiency: a failure to provide adequate oxygen to the cells of the body and to remove carbon dioxide.

Rhinitis: an inflammation of mucous membranes in the nose; the common cold.

Sore throat: pain or discomfort from inflammation of any combination of the tonsils, larynx, or pharynx; also called pharyngitis.

Tachypnea: exaggeratedly rapid breathing.

Tuberculosis: a contagious, life-threatening disease caused by a bacterial infection and spread through person-to-person contact (e.g., inhaling an infected person's sneeze).

 Tips for Passing

Don't hold your breath! That is a stress reaction, and you are depriving your brain (and the rest of your tissues) of vital oxygen. Practice breathing slowly from the diaphragm—in slowly, out slowly—and try to maintain that nice rhythm while you are taking the test.

Practice Questions

1. The study of the lungs is called
   a. Laryngology
   b. Pulmonology
   c. Orthology
   d. Otorhinolaryngology
2. The voice box is the
   a. Trachea
   b. Nasopharynx
   c. Glottis
   d. Larynx
3. The air left in the lungs after a maximum exhalation is
   a. Tidal volume
   b. Residual volume

Affirmation

My breathing is effortless.
My brain is getting all the
oxygen it needs.

    c. Bronchial volume

    d. Vital volume

4. Small sacs in the lungs that fill with air are the

    a. Bronchioles

    b. Bronchi

    c. Alveoli

    d. Epiglottis

5. The dome-shaped muscle between the thoracic and abdominal cavities that controls breathing by relaxing and contracting is the

    a. Pyramidalis

    b. Diaphragm

    c. Psoas

    d. External oblique

6. ARDS is the acronym for

    a. Alveoli residual distress syndrome

    b. Acute resting distress seizure

    c. Active respiratory disease syndrome

    d. Acute respiratory distress syndrome

7. Metabolic reactions produce an excess of _____, which must be eliminated quickly from the body.

    a. Nitrogen

    b. Mucus

    c. Carbon dioxide

    d. Perspiration

8. The larger air passages in the lungs are the

    a. Brachialis

    b. Bronchioles

    c. Bronchi

    d. Brachii

9. The exchange of gases between the air spaces in the lungs and the blood in the pulmonary capillaries is called

    a. Internal respiration

    b. External ventilation

    c. External respiration

    d. Internal ventilation

10. The trachea is commonly known as the

    a. Voice box

    b. Air filter

    c. Nasal passage

    d. Windpipe

CHAPTER 17

The Digestive System

The test of a vocation is the love of the drudgery that it involves.

—LOGAN PEARSALL SMITH

HIGHLIGHTS

The study of the digestive system is known as **gastroenterology.** The digestive system functions to take in and process food and eliminate wastes. The components of the digestive system can be discussed in terms of two categories: the gastrointestinal tract organs and the accessory organs (Fig. 17.1)

The **gastrointestinal (GI) tract,** also called the **digestive tract,** is a long system of passageways for the transit of food from the point where it is ingested to the point where waste is expelled. The organs of the GI tract are the mouth, pharynx, esophagus, stomach, small intestine, and large intestine. The **accessory organs** are the teeth, tongue, salivary glands, liver, gallbladder, and pancreas. The accessory structures and organs are not part of the GI tract.

The digestive system performs five major processes: ingestion, secretion, motility, digestion, absorption, and defecation. Food cannot be used for cellular energy until it is broken down into molecules that can cross the plasma membrane of cells; this breakdown process is called **digestion.** The passage of these molecules into the cells for use as fuel is called **absorption. Ingestion** is the act of eating or taking in liquids through the mouth. As soon as food is ingested, the process of **secretion** begins. **Salivary glands** start breaking down food by secreting **saliva. Sublingual salivary glands** are under the tongue, **submandibular salivary glands** are under the jawbone in the lower cheeks, and **parotid salivary glands** are in the upper cheeks near the ears. The **gustatory organs,** or **taste buds,** are located on the **tongue.** The **pharynx,** a structure that is also part of the respiratory system, is the cone-shaped opening at the back of the mouth that leads into the **esophagus.** The cell walls of the digestive tract secrete

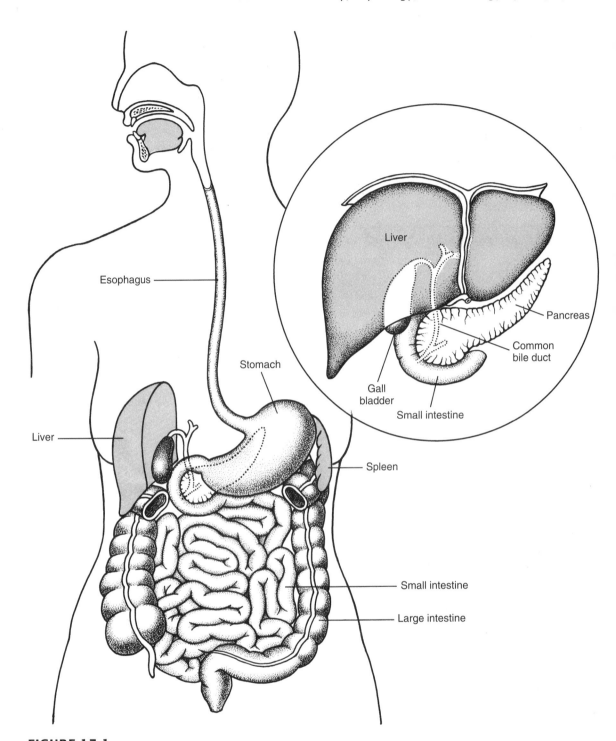

FIGURE 17.1
Components of the digestive system. (Reprinted with permission from Werner R, Benjamin BE. A Massage Therapist's Guide to Pathology, 2nd ed. Baltimore: Lippincott Williams & Wilkins. Fig. 7.1.)

enzymes, water, **acids,** and **buffers** that help break down food. **Motility** is the mixing and **propulsion** (pushing) that takes place in the GI tract through alternating contractions and relaxation of the smooth muscle walls; this rhythmic movement is also referred to as **peristalsis.** The action can be compared with a food processor—churning up the food and sending it all the way through the GI tract.

Digestion consists of two processes, mechanical digestion and chemical digestion.

Mechanical digestion is the action of the teeth grinding the food, followed by the muscles of the **stomach** and **small intestine** churning the food. After the food is dissolved and mixed with digestive enzymes and **gastric juices, chemical digestion** breaks down the larger molecules of carbohydrates, proteins, lipids, and nucleic acids into smaller molecules.

The next step in the digestive process is absorption, in which the usable digested molecules are absorbed from the GI tract and enter the bloodstream and the lymphatic system. In turn, cells absorb the molecules from the blood, where they are used for fuel, providing energy to the body systems.

The main function of the **pancreas** is the secretion of insulin and glucagon to regulate blood sugar levels; the pancreas also secretes digestive enzymes that breakdown fats and proteins in the small intestine. The liver plays a major role in metabolism, digestion, detoxification, and the elimination of wastes from the body. The **gallbladder** stores the bile produced by the liver, which breaks down and absorbs fats through the small intestine.

The digested food next passes through the **large intestine,** also called the **colon.** The large intestine is divided into six distinct parts: the **caecum, ascending colon, transverse colon, descending colon, sigmoid colon,** and **rectum.** The colon forms and stores waste matter before it is expelled from the body. The **appendix** is a sac-like organ projecting from the caecum at the beginning of the colon. We don't really know the function of the appendix; although it is attached to the digestive system, it does not seem to have an active role there and may in fact be part of the immune system.

The final digestive process is **defecation,** the elimination of waste products that have not been absorbed by the body. Defecation takes place through the **anus,** the opening at the rectum. The waste products are referred to as **feces.**

Each of the food groups we consume has different nutritional value for the healthy functioning of the body. **Carbohydrates** are sugars and starches that fuel the body. They provide the energy to meet our immediate needs for physical activity and brain function. Carbohydrates are found in starchy vegetables, fruits, and some grains. **Proteins** are made from 20 amino acids (Table 17.1).Proteins act as enzymes, hormones, and **immunoglobins,** which are **antibodies** vital to immunological function. Proteins are involved in oxygen transport, electrical impulses, muscle contraction, and many other functions in the body. They provide energy from foods such as meat, fish, fowl, dairy products, and some nuts and grains. Of the 20 amino acids, 10 are considered to be "essential," meaning that they must be provided in the diet because the body cannot make them. The other 10 are referred to as "nonessential" because the body is capable of manufacturing them.

Nucleic acids include **DNA (deoxyribonucleic acid)** and **RNA (ribonucleic acid). Lipids** are what we usually think of as fats, but they can also be steroids and waxes (ear wax is a lipid). Lipids store energy for the body; as body fat, they also cushion internal organs and provide insulation. Lipids are obtained from plant and animal sources. **Cholesterol,** which is a lipid, comes only from animal sources such as meat, eggs, and dairy foods.

WHAT YOU NEED TO KNOW

Absorption: the process of absorbing substances into cells or across tissues.

Alimentary canal: another term for the GI tract (digestive tract).

Anus: the terminal opening of the GI tract.

TABLE 17.1 Amino Acids

Amino Acids	Main Functions	Food Source
Alanine	Breaks down glucose (sugar)	Mainly meats
Arginine	Aids body during stress or injury and acts as growth hormone	Mainly turkey, poultry, other meats
Asparagine	Assists in metabolic functioning of brain cells and nervous system cells	Legumes, many other foods
Aspartic acid	Expels ammonia from body, helps immune functions	Legumes, many other food
Cysteine	Collagen production, immune functions	Wheat, poultry, broccoli, onions, garlic, peppers
Glutamine	Brain function, muscle function and repair	Fish, meat, beans, dairy, spinach parsley
Glutamic acid	Important excitatory neurotransmitter; helps metabolize sugar and fat	Meat, poultry, fish, eggs
Glycine	Simplest amino acid; regulates calcium; major inhibitory neurotransmitter	Fish, meat, beans, dairy
Histidine	Immune functions; nerve tissue growth and repair, especially myelin sheath; involved in blood cell production	Dairy, meat, poultry, fish, rye, wheat, rice
Isoleucine	Red blood cell production, blood's ability to clot, muscle recovery after strenuous exercise	Almonds, cashews, chicken, liver, eggs, fish
Leucine	Blood sugar regulation, musculoskeletal support, helps manage stress	All protein foods
Lysine	Growth and bone development in children; calcium absorption; maintains correct nitrogen balance in body; produce antibodies, hormones, enzymes; collagen formation as well as tissue repair	Most protein foods
Methionine	Breaks down fats; antioxidant	Meat, beans, yogurt, lentils, garlic, seeds
Phenylalanine	Needed to synthesize dopamine and norepinephrine	Almonds, avocados, lima beans, nuts and seeds, dairy, and meat
Proline	Produces collagen; skin renewal	Most protein foods

continued

TABLE 17.1	Amino Acids *(Continued)*	
Amino Acids	**Main Functions**	**Food Source**
Serine	Fat metabolism, tissue growth, immune system functions	Wheat, dairy, meats
Threonine	Maintains protein balance, collagen and elastin production, liver function	Meat, dairy, eggs, some vegetables
Tryptophan	Needed for production of niacin and serotonin, nerve and brain function	Cottage cheese, meat, soy protein
Tyrosine	Needed to produce neurotransmitters	Meat, dairy, eggs, bananas, avocados
Valine	Muscle metabolism, maintains nitrogen balance in body	Dairy, meat, grain mushrooms

Ascending colon: the first section of the large intestine, beginning in the lower right quadrant of the abdomen and ending in the upper right quadrant at the transverse colon.

Bile: a yellow–green liquid substance secreted by the liver that aids in the absorption of fats; stored in the gallbladder.

Chyme: food that has been acted upon by digestive enzymes but has not yet passed into the small intestine.

Common bile duct: a duct that transports bile from the liver and gallbladder to the duodenum.

Cystic duct: the duct that connects the common bile duct to the gallbladder.

Descending colon: the fourth segment of the large intestine that connects the transverse colon to the sigmoid colon.

Duodenum: the first segment of the small intestine connecting the pylorus and the jejunum.

Esophagus: the segment of the digestive tract between the pharynx and the stomach.

External anal sphincter: a ring of striated muscle fibers surrounding the anal opening.

Fundus: the bottom of any hollow organ, such as the stomach.

Gallbladder: the organ that stores the bile that is produced in the liver; involved in the absorption of fats.

Gastric juice: the liquid secretions of the stomach.

Gingivae: the gums of the mouth.

Greater omentum: part of the peritoneum, the sac that covers most of the intestines.

Ileocecal valve: the entryway to the colon from the small intestine.

Ileum: the last segment of the small intestine connecting with the large intestine.

Internal anal sphincter: the ring of smooth muscle surrounding the internal part of the anal opening.

Jejunum: the segment of the small intestine connecting the duodenum to the ileum.

Large intestine: the digestive organ that forms and transports waste matter from the rest of the GI tract. In the human adult, it is approximately 5 feet long. Also called colon.

Lesser omentum: part of the peritoneum that connects the stomach and liver.

Liver: a digestive organ in the upper right quadrant of the abdomen that plays a major role in metabolism, digestion, and elimination.

Mastication: the process of chewing food.

Mesentery: the membrane that connects the intestines to the abdominal wall.

Mesocolon: the fold of the peritoneum that is attached to the colon.

Mucosa: the mucous membrane lining the GI tract.

Muscularis: the muscular inner coating of the GI tract.

Pancreas: a small organ that lies behind the stomach and secretes powerful digestive enzymes into the small bowel as well as the hormones that regulate blood sugar (insulin and glucagon).

Parotid salivary glands: salivary glands in front of and inferior to the ear.

Peritoneum: the smooth membrane that lines the abdomen. It folds back over the organs, at which point it is referred to as the visceral peritoneum.

Pyloric sphincter: the thick muscular valve that allows food to move into the duodenum.

Pylorus: the opening from the stomach to the intestine.

Rectum: the last segment of the large intestine that joins the sigmoid colon and the anus.

Rugae: the folds of the gastric mucosa (stomach lining).

Saliva: the secretions of the salivary glands.

Salivary glands: glands that produce saliva to moisten the oral cavity and food; saliva contains antibodies and other substances that protect against infections in the mouth as well as enzymes that aid in the digestion of carbohydrates.

Serosa: delicate membranes that line the internal cavities of the body.

Sigmoid colon: the segment of the colon that connects the descending colon to the rectum.

Small intestine: the tube of the GI tract with three distinct segments (duodenum, jejunum, and ileum) that are involved in the absorption of nutrients into the body. In the human adult, it is approximately 22 feet long.

Stomach: the largest portion of the GI tract, situated between the esophagus and the small intestine; it secretes gastric juices to assist in the breakdown of food.

Sublingual salivary glands: salivary glands located under the tongue.

Submandibular salivary glands: salivary glands located under the jawbone.

Submucosa: the layer of tissue beneath a mucous membrane.

Teeth: the hard appendages in the mouth made of dentine and enamel that enable mastication (chewing).

Uvula: the tear-shaped appendage hanging down in the center of the edge of the soft palate.

Villi: tiny projections on the inner intestine walls that aid in absorption.

PATHOLOGY OF THE DIGESTIVE SYSTEM

The pathology of the digestive system encompasses many conditions, from a simple stomach ache to cancer. Because food goes in one end and comes out the other, there is a lot of biological terrain in between and opportunity for things to go wrong. The food we eat (and how much of it) has everything to do with the health of our digestive system. How much water we consume also is vital to good digestive health. **Stress** plays a major role in many dysfunctions of the digestive system; **peptic ulcers, acid reflux,** and **irritable bowel syndrome (IBS)** are just a few examples of conditions that can be caused or aggravated by stress.

Poor nutrition can affect many bodily functions. Obesity is a direct cause of or contributor to many illnesses elsewhere in the body. **Malabsorption** and **intolerance disorders** occur whenever the system is unable to absorb a vital nutrient or tolerate a specific substance. **Cystic fibrosis** is not thought of as a digestive disorder, but it has a major relationship with digestion in that it causes pancreatic and liver dysfunction as well as electrolyte dysfunction. **Bowel obstruction** prohibits the passage of food through the intestines and may be life-threatening if not treated. **Constipation** and **diarrhea** are two consequences of bowel obstruction; diarrhea would seem to be the opposite of obstructed, but the fact is there is usually constipation present and the liquid fecal matter is the only thing passing through.

Hemorrhoids are red and painful dilated blood vessels around the opening of the anus that often accompany constipation and/or diarrhea.

Appendicitis is an inflammation of the **appendix.**

Although **anorexia nervosa** and **bulimia nervosa** are actually psychological disorders, they are also eating disorders and therefore related to the digestive system. Many illnesses that originate in other body systems have some effect on the digestive system—and digestive disorders can affect all other body systems.

Achalasia: a constriction in the lower portion of the esophagus caused by unrelaxed sphincter muscles.

Acid reflux: the abnormal return of stomach contents back into the esophagus; also called gastroesophageal reflux disease (GERD) if chronic, or reflux esophagitis.

Adhesion: fibrous bands abnormally binding to tissue (such as scar tissue).

Anorexia nervosa: an eating disorder characterized by an unrealistic self-image of the body, with a pathological fear of becoming fat, excessive dieting, and emaciation. No loss of appetite occurs until the late stages of the disease; primarily affects girls and young women.

Appendicitis: an inflammation of the appendix.

Borborygmus: "rumbling" noises in the GI tract, caused by gas moving through the intestines.

Bulimia nervosa: an eating disorder characterized by self-induced purging (vomiting and/or diuretic and laxative abuse) after binge eating; strict dieting, fasting, or obsessive exercising to prevent weight gain.

Canker sore: a small, painful crater in the mouth; also called an aphthous ulcer.

Cholecystitis: an inflammation of the gallbladder.

Cirrhosis of the liver: the loss of healthy tissue accompanied by fibrosis and chronic inflammation.

Colitis: an inflammation of the colon.

Colostomy: the surgical construction of an artificial opening of the colon through the abdominal wall as a treatment for serious digestive problems.

Constipation: difficulty in eliminating feces.

Crohn's disease: chronic inflammation of the digestive or GI tract.

Diarrhea: overly frequent and loose or fluid evacuations of the large intestine.

Diverticulitis: an inflammation of a sac-like appendage on the inside walls of the large intestine.

Dysphagia: difficulty in swallowing.

Enteritis: an inflammation of the small intestine.

Femoral hernia: a mass in the groin stemming from a looped large intestine that occurs most frequently in overweight females.

Flatus: digestive gas.

Gallbladder disease: a chronic inflammation of the gallbladder, usually accompanied by gallstones.

Gastritis: an inflammation of the stomach.

Gastroenteritis: an acute inflammation of the lining of the GI tract.

Gingivitis: an inflammation of the gums.

Heartburn: indigestion accompanied by a burning sensation.

Hepatitis A: a generally non-life threatening disease that is transmitted through contaminated food and drink and causes flu-like symptoms after a 2-week incubation period.

Hepatitis B: a viral disease, spread by contact with contaminated blood or passed through the placenta from mother to child; a person can be a carrier and be asymptomatic; severe infections are characteristic, as is cirrhosis of the liver. Also called serum hepatitis.

Hepatitis C: a viral disease most commonly caused through the transfusion of infected blood; spreading by sexual contact is rare. The signs and symptoms are very similar to that of hepatitis B.

Hernia: a protrusion of an organ through the body wall or into another organ, such as a loop of the large intestine protruding through the abdomen.

Hiatal hernia: a type of hernia in which part of the stomach is protruding through the diaphragm.

Inflammatory bowel disease (IBD): name of a group of disorders that cause inflammation in the intestines.

Irritable bowel syndrome (IBS): a chronic condition of the large intestine, characterized by recurrent abdominal cramps and diarrhea, often alternating with periods of constipation; usually attributed to stress.

Jaundice: a yellowing of the skin and the whites of the eyes, caused by a buildup of a bile pigment.

Malnutrition: inadequate nutrition, but not the same thing as starvation. A person could eat three meals per day and still have malnutrition.

Nausea: a queasy feeling in the GI tract or general abdomen, often culminating in vomiting.

Obesity: excessive fat in the body.

Peptic ulcer: an ulcer in the esophagus, stomach, or proximal small intestine, caused by gastric juices eating through the mucous membrane.

Vomiting: regurgitation of the stomach contents.

Tips for Passing

Use the definitions in sentences: "Yellow skin is a sign of jaundice." Repetition!

Practice Questions

1. The study of the digestive system is known as
   a. Gastroenterology
   b. Intestinology
   c. Tractology
   d. Endology

2. Bile is secreted by the
   a. Stomach
   b. Colon
   c. Gallbladder
   d. Liver

3. The adult large intestine is approximately _____ feet in length.
   a. 2
   b. 5
   c. 10
   d. 22

4. Mastication is
   a. Surgical removal of the breast
   b. An opening in the stomach lining
   c. The process of chewing food
   d. Part of the upper jawbone

5. The opening from the stomach to the intestine is the
   a. Rectum
   b. Pylorus
   c. Bile duct
   d. Parotid gland

6. The organ that secretes insulin is the
   a. Pancreas
   b. Gallbladder
   c. Liver
   d. Thyroid

7. Gingivae is (are)
   a. A bacterial infection
   b. Small openings in the back of the throat
   c. The gums of the mouth
   d. A connection between the large and small intestines

8. Part of the stomach protruding through the diaphragm is a(n)
   a. Colostomy
   b. Hiatal hernia
   c. Colonoscopy
   d. Peptic ulcer

Affirmation

I am equal to the task.

9. Binge eating and purging are known as
   a. Anorexia
   b. Bulimia necrosa
   c. Amaryllis nervosa
   d. Bulimia nervosa

10. Borborygmus is caused by
    a. Difficulty absorbing potassium
    b. Gas moving through the intestines
    c. Frequent urination
    d. Cirrhosis of the liver

CHAPTER **18**

The Urinary System

Having intelligence is not as important as knowing when to use it, just as having a hoe is not as important as knowing when to plant.

—ANCIENT CHINESE PROVERB

HIGHLIGHTS

The urinary system can be thought of as the body's water treatment plant. The main structures of the urinary system include two kidneys, two ureters, the urinary bladder, and the urethra (Fig. 18.1). The functions of the urinary system are to filter blood and to regulate blood volume and blood pressure. This body system manages blood composition, including maintaining pH to prevent blood plasma from becoming too acidic or basic by regulating ions; it regulates hormone levels in the blood, maintains water balance in the body, and facilitates the excretion of wastes through the urine.

The study of the urinary system (and in males, the reproductive system also) is known as **urology.** In males, the urethra is also the tube that carries semen on its way out of the body, as well as urine, so there is overlap among the two systems.

The **kidneys** are bean-shaped organs located in the posterior abdominal cavity on either side of the spinal column. They are the main filtering plant of the urinary system. The kidneys produce **erythropoietin,** which stimulates red blood cell synthesis, and **renin,** which helps control salt and water balance and blood pressure. They are also involved in regulating plasma volume to ensure an adequate quantity to keep blood flowing to vital organs. The kidneys help keep extracellular fluid from becoming too dilute or concentrated, and they maintain relatively constant levels of key **ions,** including sodium, potassium, and calcium.

The kidneys are attached to the posterior abdominal wall and surrounded by three layers of tissue: the **renal capsule,** the **adipose capsule,** and **renal fascia.** Blood flows

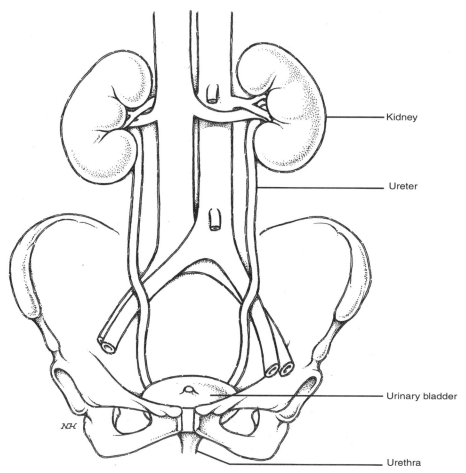

FIGURE 18.1
The female urinary tract. (Adapted with permission from Neil O. Hardy, Westpoint, CT.)

into the kidneys through the **renal arteries** and works its way through the different structures within the kidneys before flowing out through the **renal veins.**

The study of the kidneys is known as **nephrology.** The workhorses of the kidneys, the **nephrons,** perform three basic functions: filtration, secretion, and reabsorption. Each kidney has about a million nephrons. The nephrons are **tubules** (tiny tubes) originating on the outer layer of the kidney, the **renal cortex,** ending in a collecting tubule, which then empties into the renal pelvis to which the ureter is connected, and eventually merging to empty into the urinary bladder. The tubule opening of the nephron where water and solutes empty from the bloodstream is called **Bowman's capsule.** The fluid then flows through the proximal tubule before dipping into the **loop of Henle,** or **nephron loop.** The loop of Henle then goes downward to the center of the kidney, the **renal medulla,** before rising back up to the cortex. The **distal convoluted tubule** remains in the cortex, and multiple tubules combine at the **collecting tubule** to descend together to the medulla. The two adrenal glands are located above each kidney and are thus sometimes referred to as suprarenal glands, but they are part of the endocrine system, not the urinary system. An overview of the urinary system is shown in Figure 18.2.

During this filtration, up to 180 liters per day pass through the **glomerulus,** a network of capillaries inside the Bowman's capsule; only approximately 1.5 liters per

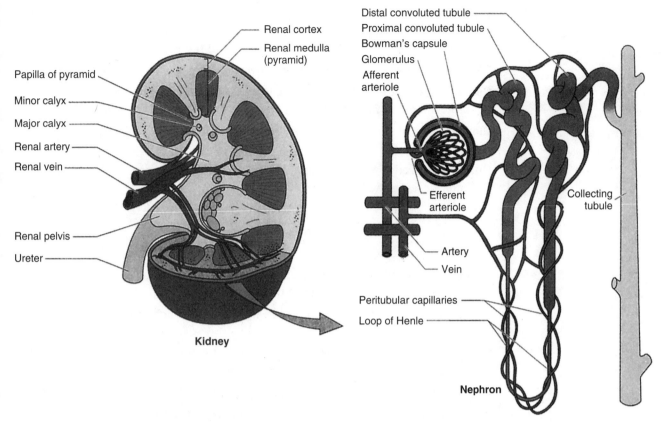

FIGURE 18.2
Overview of the urinary system. (Reprinted with permission from Willis MC, Medical Terminology: The Language of Health Care. Baltimore: Williams & Wilkins, 1996:407.)

day are expelled as urine. Most substances pass through easily, but blood cells and proteins are not usually filtered. Substances that are not needed by the body are removed and discharged into the **urine** through a process known as **tubular secretion.** Substances that can be utilized by the body are maintained through **reabsorption.** Normally, urine is approximately 95% water and 5% solutes that the body cannot use. The kidneys have a large functional reserve. It is possible to lose 75% of the nephrons' capacity and still maintain homeostasis. Thus, the body can function on one kidney.

The **ureters** transport urine from the kidneys to the **urinary bladder,** a hollow organ that holds urine before it is released as waste via the **urethra.** When the bladder is empty, it is collapsed; it regains its shape only as it fills with urine, which is an ongoing process, because the kidneys are constantly filtering. The excretion of urine occurs when the bladder contracts and the internal and external sphincters relax to allow the passage of urine out of the body.

WHAT YOU NEED TO KNOW

Afferent arteriole: a small vessel that conveys blood to the glomerulus.

Bowman's capsule: the tubule opening of the nephron where water and solutes empty from the bloodstream.

Calyx: inlet on the renal pelvis where urine is collected from the renal pyramids. Plural: calyces.

Convoluted tubule: twisted segments of the nephrons on either side of the loop of Henle. The proximal convoluted tubule is the first segment of the nephron; the distal convoluted tubule is the last segment of the nephron.

Efferent arteriole: a small vessel that conveys blood away from the glomerulus.

Glomerular filtration rate: a measurement of the kidney's ability to filter and remove waste products from the blood.

Glomerulus: a network of capillaries inside the Bowman's capsule involved in filtering blood.

Hilus: the curved area of the kidney where the renal artery, renal vein, and ureters enter or leave the kidney.

Kidney: one of the two large bean-shaped organs that are the main filters of blood.

Loop of Henle: the U-shaped part of a nephron.

Micturition: urination.

Nephron: the small filtering unit in the kidney made up of blood vessels and tubules; it is the working unit of the kidney.

Papilla: a projection that has small openings through which urine drains out of the nephron.

Peritubular capillary: a vessel arising from the efferent arteriole that runs alongside and around the renal tubules and drains into the renal venous system.

Renal capsule: fibrous connective tissue surrounding the kidneys.

Renal medulla: the center of the kidney, where the renal pyramids are located.

Renal pelvis: the extension of the ureters inside the kidney that collects urine from the calyces and sends it down the ureters.

Renal pyramid: a triangular area in the kidney that contains nephrons.

Ureter: one of two tubes that transport urine from the kidneys to the urinary bladder.

Urethra: the tube that transports urine from the urinary bladder to the outside of the body.

Urinary bladder: the sac that holds urine before it is expelled from the body; urination occurs when the bladder contracts.

Urine: the liquid waste excreted from the kidneys.

PATHOLOGY OF THE URINARY SYSTEM

Because the urinary system is the body's filtering system, serious problems can potentially affect all other systems. The most serious affliction of the urinary system is **kidney disease,** a general term for a number of chronic conditions causing damage to the kidneys. **Chronic kidney failure** is an irreversible and progressive wasting of the kidneys that causes serious interference with metabolic functioning. The only treatments are dialysis (until death) or kidney transplant. **Dialysis** is a method of filtering the blood by artificial means outside the body and returning it to the circulation.

Urine sometimes contains abnormal substances or unusual amounts of substances that would normally be present. **Kidney stones,** or **renal calculi,** are crystallized secretions composed of calcium, phosphates, or urea. They are usually passed during urination but in severe cases may have to be medically treated or surgically removed. **Glucosuria** is the presence of glucose (sugar) in the urine. Glucose does filter into the urine, but the kidneys normally reabsorb all of the glucose and put it back into the blood. However, if blood sugars become too high, such as during diabetes, the kidneys are unable to reabsorb all the glucose, and glucose remains in the urine.

Red blood cells appearing in the urine usually are a sign of inflammation or trauma from injury, but they can also be a sign of a tumor. The appearance of **white blood cells** in abnormal amounts in the urine usually is a sign of infection anywhere in the urinary system and is referred to as **pyuria,** meaning "pus in the system." **Albumin** in the urine indicates damaged nephrons and may also mean liver damage. Some popular diets have followers checking their urine on a test strip with the intent of achieving **ketosis,** the presence of **ketones** in the urine. Because high ketone levels cause an acidic condition in the body that can lead to coma or death, it is a dangerous way to diet. This is the same condition that occurs when a diabetic subject does not take insulin. Urine that is cloudy, colored strangely, or extremely smelly can be a sign of a bladder infection or more serious diseases.

Not all urinary tract diseases occur in the kidneys. **Bladder diverticulum** is a sac-like pouch that protrudes from the bladder wall where some of the lining has been punched out, much like a hernia. It may be symptomless and not cause any problems, and some people are born with the condition. If it becomes too large, it may become a repository for urine that can become stagnated and cause an infection. **Bladder fistula** is a relatively rare condition that occurs when the bladder is abnormally attached to another organ, usually the vagina or the large intestine. Bladder fistula causes frequent bladder infections and causes gas to be passed from the urethra during urination. **Neurogenic bladder** is interference with normal bladder function caused by a spinal cord injury or a disorder affecting the autonomic nervous system, such as multiple sclerosis or diabetes. The main symptom of neurogenic bladder is incontinence.

A **urinary tract infection (UTI)** can occur anywhere in the system. Normally, urine is sterile, containing no bacteria, viruses, or fungi. Infection occurs when microorganisms, such as bacteria from the GI tract, settle at the opening of the urethra and start multiplying. Most infections are caused by the bacterium *Escherichia coli,* which normally lives in the colon.

Bacteria usually begin to grow in the urethra. An infection in the urethra is called **urethritis.** If the bacteria move to the bladder, it will become infected, a condition known as **cystitis.** If not treated promptly, bacteria will then move up through the ureters to infect the kidneys; this condition is called **pyelonephritis.** *Chlamydia* and *Mycoplasma* are other bacteria that can cause UTIs in both men and women. (The bacterium *Chlamydia trachomatis* causes a form of urethritis.) Unlike *E. coli,* these organisms can be sexually transmitted.

The urinary system functions to help ward off infection. The ureters and urinary bladder normally prevent urine from backing up, but malfunctions sometime occur. Women get UTIs more frequently than do men because their urethra is shorter and because it opens at the vagina and near the anus, two moist places where bacteria can thrive. Several factors can contribute to urinary tract infections. IUDs (intrauterine devices used for contraception) and even tampons may irritate the urinary tract. Sexual intercourse may also cause UTIs in some women. Men who are not circumcised get UTIs more frequently than men who are. UTIs are also common in hospital patients who have to have a catheter inserted and in people with a compromised immune system.

Nutrition plays an important role in the health of the urinary system. Some foods and beverages can cause the bladder muscle to contract, resulting in the strong urge to urinate with abnormal frequency. Citrus fruits and other foods high in acid, like tomatoes and cranberries, can cause bladder contractions, as can spicy foods such as Mexican, Cajun, or Thai food. Alcohol and caffeine products, such as coffee, tea, colas, and chocolate, all act as diuretics and cause excessive urination. Of all the culprits flowing through the urinary system, colas are probably the worst. Colas contain excessive sugar or artificial sweeteners, phosphoric acid, caramel coloring or other food dyes, caffeine, carbon dioxide, and aluminum. Carbon dioxide is a waste product expelled by our body with every exhalation, so why would anyone want to drink it? Phosphoric acid is a strong acid that upsets the balance between calcium and phosphorus in the blood and makes the pH very acidic. It causes excess amounts of calcium to be lost in the urine. As the body compensates for the lost calcium, osteoporosis, osteoarthritis, gout, bone spurs, bursitis, bunions, kidney stones, and other problems may result. Caffeine elevates blood pressure and heart rate, in addition to causing excessive urination, and is an addictive substance as well. Drinking adequate water helps ensure that the urinary system will function optimally.

Acute renal failure: a sudden decline in renal function.

Azotemia: an excess amount of nitrogenous waste products in the blood.

Chronic renal failure: a gradual decline in renal function.

Cystitis: an inflammation of the urinary bladder.

Cystocele: a protrusion of the urinary bladder into the vaginal canal, resulting in incontinence.

Dialysis: a mechanical filtering of the blood done as a treatment for kidney failure.

Enuresis: incontinence, including bed-wetting.

Glomerulonephritis: an inflammation of the capillary loops in the nephrons; an autoimmune disease.

Ketosis: the presence of ketones, a metabolic by-product of fat metabolism that can create a life-threatening condition. In a diabetic subject it indicates an absence of insulin.

Lithotripsy: a nonsurgical blasting of kidney stones with sound waves to break them up.

Nephritis: an inflammation of the nephrons of the kidney.

Nephrotic syndrome: an inflammation caused by an excess amount of proteins in the urine, resulting in edema.

Nocturia: Frequent night-time urination.

Polycystic kidney disease: a rare genetic condition in which the kidneys contain many cysts, resulting in chronic kidney failure usually in late middle age.

Pyelonephritis: an inflammation of the kidney caused by a bacterial infection.

Renal calculus: a kidney stone.

Renal stricture: a narrowing of any of the renal tubes.

Urethritis: an inflammation of the urethra.

Urinary retention: an inability to urinate or failure to empty the bladder totally, bladder pressure being unable to overcome urethral resistance. It can be caused by a weak bladder wall or urethral obstruction.

Urinary tract infection (UTI): an inflammation of any of the structures of the urinary system.

Urolithiasis: another name for kidney stones.

Tips for Passing

Understand that a lapse in memory is a perfectly normal occurrence, and don't stress out over it. Leave that question and come back to it later.

Practice Questions

1. The sac that holds urine before it is expelled from the body is the
   a. Kidney
   b. Gallbladder
   c. Urinary bladder
   d. Nephron

2. There are _____ ureters in the body.
   a. 1
   b. 2
   c. 3
   d. 4

3. In males, the tube that carries semen on its way out of the body is the
   a. Prostate
   b. Urethra
   c. Ureter
   d. Fallopian tube

4. Renal calculi are
   a. Tubes leaving the nephron
   b. Factors that cause a hardening of the kidneys
   c. Kidney stones
   d. Urinary tract infections

5. The tubes that transport urine from the kidneys to the bladder are the
   a. Bowman's capsules
   b. Ureters
   c. Urethras
   d. Renal capsules

6. Metabolic byproducts of fat metabolism are
   a. Enzymes
   b. Ketones
   c. Vitamin A
   d. Norephrenine

7. A mechanical filtering of the blood to treat kidney failure is called
   a. Renalysis
   b. Nephrolysis
   c. Urethrasis
   d. Dialysis

8. An excessive amount of nitrogenous waste products in the blood is known as
   a. Nitrogena
   b. Toxemia
   c. Azotemia
   d. Enuresis

Affirmation

I live in the present. Past failures are unimportant.

9. Frequent night-time urination is referred to as
   a. Nephrotic syndrome
   b. Catherization
   c. Nocturia
   d. Catharsis

10. The structures of the urinary system are the
    a. Kidneys, ureters, urinary bladder, urethra
    b. Kidneys, prostate, urinary bladder, urethra
    c. Kidneys, ureters, urinary bladder, gall bladder
    d. Kidneys, ureters, urinary bladder, bowels

CHAPTER 19

The Reproductive System

O this learning, what a thing it is!

—WILLIAM SHAKESPEARE

HIGHLIGHTS

The structures of the reproductive system are different in males and females. The **gonads** are the ovaries in females and the testes in males; they produce egg cells and sperm cells, which are known as **gametes.**

The female reproductive structures include the ovaries, the uterus, the Fallopian tubes, the vagina, and the external genitals, referred to as the vulva. Major structures of the female reproductive system are shown in Figure 19.1. The **mammary glands,** or breasts, secrete milk during the process of **lactation** and are also part of the female reproductive system. The **ovaries** are two oval structures located on each side of the uterus where the egg cells develop and are released during **ovulation.** The eggs travel down the **Fallopian tubes** to the **uterus,** a hollow organ approximately 3 inches long in a nonpregnant woman. During pregnancy, a fertilized egg becomes embedded in the uterus, which houses the **embryo** until birth, a period of approximately 40 weeks known as **gestation.**

Pregnancy is divided into three **trimesters** that represent different phases in the development of the **fetus.** At the end of the third trimester, the woman goes into **labor** and delivers the newborn. The baby is delivered through the **vagina,** or **birth canal,** which is also the female sex organ.

Labor occurs in three stages: dilation, expulsion, and the placental stage. During **dilation,** the uterine opening, called the **cervix,** dilates to accommodate the passage of the baby through the birth canal—the act of **expulsion.** During the third stage **(placental stage),** the **placenta,** a special tissue within the uterus that houses the baby and amniotic fluid during pregnancy, is expelled a short time after the baby is born.

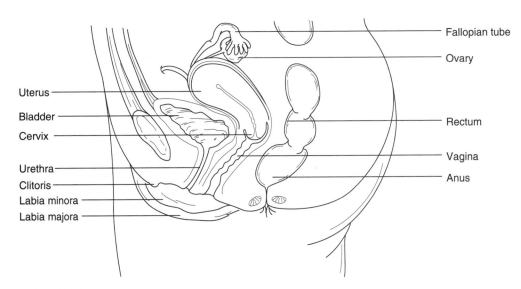

FIGURE 19.1
The female reproductive system. (Reprinted with permission from Ashton J, Cassel D. Review for Therapeutic Massage and Bodywork Certification. Baltimore: Lippincott Williams & Wilkins, 2002:89. Fig. 16.2.)

The **amniotic fluid** cushions the baby from injury and is important to fetal development. Parental bonding will, in normal circumstances, take place almost immediately as parents and child meet each other for the first time.

The **vulva** is the external opening of the vagina. It is composed of two pairs of lips, the **labia majora** (larger) and **labia minora** (smaller). At the top of the vagina is a small mass of erect tissue, the **clitoris.** The opening of the vagina is called the **vestibule.** The **vestibular glands** secrete mucus during sexual arousal. The smallest part of the opening is the **vaginal orifice.** The **mons pubis** is the padding of fatty tissue that covers the pubic symphysis (the pubic bone).

Females have a **menstrual cycle.** At the time of **puberty,** or sexual maturity, young women begin **menstruation,** the monthly sloughing off of the **endometrium,** the uterine lining, as a bloody discharge. The onset of menstruation is referred to as **menarche.** Monthly bleeding, referred to as the **menstrual period,** continues for approximately 40 years, unless it is interrupted by an abnormality, pregnancy, or a pharmaceutical or surgical intervention. During puberty, the **secondary sex characteristics,** the growth of breasts and public hair, also occurs. Usually during their fifties, women cease menstruating, a phase called **menopause.**

The male reproductive structures include the testes, epididymis, vas deferens, ejaculatory duct, urethra, seminal vesicles, prostate gland, bulbourethral glands, and the penis (Fig. 19.2). The **epididymis** is a structure that stores sperm and is the place where sperm **motility** (motion) increases. It is tightly coiled into approximately 1.5 inches, but if it were straightened out, it would be approximately 20 feet long. The **vas deferens** also stores sperm, and the sperm can remain viable there for months. Sperm cells that are not ejaculated are reabsorbed by the body. The **ejaculatory ducts** pass through the **prostate gland,** where they eject sperm and other seminal secretions just before ejaculation through the penis. Two **seminal vesicles,** located behind the urinary bladder and above the prostate, contribute fluid to the ejaculate. The **penis,** the male sex organ, has a **root,** a **body,** and an **extremity,** which is also called the **glans.** The root is attached to the pubic bone. The **corpora cavernosa** runs the length of the penis

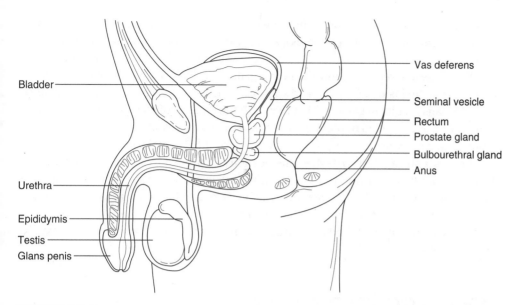

FIGURE 19.2
The male reproductive system. (Reprinted with permission from Ashton J, Cassel D. Review for Therapeutic Massage and Bodywork Certification. Baltimore: Lippincott Williams & Wilkins, 2002:88. Fig. 16.1.)

and has two spaces filled with spongy tissue. During sexual arousal, blood rushes to the spaces in the spongy tissue and causes an **erection.** The **corpus spongiosum** lies under the corpora cavernosa and houses the urethra as it descends.

The glans of the penis is covered in a mucous membrane and a **prepuce,** or **foreskin,** if the male has not undergone **circumcision.** The **urethra** in males serves as the passageway for both urine and semen as it is expelled from the body. The **bulbourethral glands,** also known as **Cowper's glands,** secrete mucus that lubricates the penis and the lining of the urethra, and during sexual arousal also secretes an alkaline substance that neutralizes the uric acids in the urethra, so sperm can pass through undamaged. The **testes,** or **testicles,** which produce sperm, are housed in a pouch-like sac called the **scrotum.**

During puberty, young men start to grow pubic and facial hair, and their voice deepens. Adolescent males may also experience nocturnal erection and ejaculation. In both sexes, **libido,** or sexual desire, comes into consciousness during puberty.

The function of the reproductive system is **sexual reproduction,** the process of creating offspring, through the union of male and female gametes. When a **sperm cell,** the male gamete, unites with an **egg cell,** or **ovum, fertilization** takes place, and barring a medical emergency or an abortion, offspring will be the result. The branch of medicine dealing with the female reproductive system is known as **gynecology.** The branch of medicine that deals specifically with pregnancy, childbirth, and the period during recovery from childbirth is known as **obstetrics.** The branch of medicine dealing with the male reproductive systems falls under **urology,** which also includes the study of the urinary system.

Human cells contain 23 pairs of chromosomes, called **homologous chromosomes,** that contain the same gene sequences; one chromosome from each pair is inherited from each parent. Every person has one pair of chromosomes known as **sex chromosomes,** referred to as X and Y chromosomes. In females, the homologous sex chromosomes are both X chromosomes; in males, they are one X and one Y. The remaining

22 pairs are referred to as **autosomes. Somatic cells** are all the cells of the body other than the reproductive cells (gametes), such as kidney cells, brain cells, liver cells, and so on. They contain two sets of chromosomes and are referred to as **diploid cells.**

During sexual reproduction, the new organism, a single diploid cell called a **zygote,** results from the fusion of the egg and sperm, a process called **conception.** Cell division in the gonads results in gametes that have half the number of chromosomes of somatic cells. Gametes are called **haploid cells** because they contain only a single set of chromosomes, caused by specialized cell division, referred to as **meiosis.**

Contraception refers to devices, medications, or procedures to prevent pregnancy. Examples are IUDs (intrauterine devices), birth control pills, the "morning after" pill, and spermicides. The rhythm method, which is avoiding intercourse when the woman is ovulating, is the least reliable method of birth control but still used by some women. Condoms are the only method of contraception that provides protection from **sexually transmitted diseases (STDs).**

WHAT YOU NEED TO KNOW

Amniotic fluid: the serous fluid within the placenta that cushions the baby from injury; important to fetal development.

Areola: a circle of dark-colored skin around the nipple.

Autosome: a chromosome that is not a sex chromosome.

Breasts: the female mammary glands, which produce milk.

Chromosome: a genetic structure of the cell that carries the DNA.

Clitoris: a small mass of erect tissue at the entrance to the vagina; homologous to the penis in males; can give a woman sexual pleasure when touched.

Diploid cell: a cell containing all the genetic material.

Ejaculation: the expulsion of semen.

Endometrium: the lining of the uterus that is expelled during the menstrual period and grows back each cycle.

Fallopian tubes: tubes that transport egg cells from the ovaries to the womb.

Gametes: egg cells and sperm cells.

Gonads: the ovaries in females, the testes in males.

Labia majora: the outer pair of lips of the vulva, the external female genitals.

Labia minora: the inner pair of lips of the vulva, the external female genitals.

Mammary glands: the milk-producing glands in females; the breasts.

Meiosis: a type of cell division that occurs in two successive divisions that results in haploid cells.

Menarche: the onset of menstruation.

Menopause: the gradual decline and ultimate cessation of the menstrual cycle.

Menstrual cycle: the reproductive cycle, characterized by the monthly discharge of blood from the uterus.

Myometrium: a smooth muscle of the uterus.

Ovaries: two small bean-shaped female gonads where eggs are developed and released.

Ovum: an egg cell.

Penis: the male sex organ, where urine is also expelled.

Perimetrium: a thin fluid coating of the uterus.

Placenta: a special tissue within the uterus that houses the baby and amniotic fluid during pregnancy; it joins the mother to her fetus and provides the fetus with oxygen, water, and nutrients from the mother's blood and secretes the hormones necessary for a successful pregnancy.

Prostate gland: a gland in males surrounding the neck of the urinary bladder and urethra that aids in the manufacture of semen.

Puberty: the period during which sexual reproduction becomes possible, usually during early adolescence, and during which secondary sex characteristics, such as breasts in females, a lower voice in males, and pubic hair in both sexes, begin to develop.

Scrotum: a sac that houses the testicles.

Semen: the fluid released during ejaculation that contains sperm and secretions from the prostate gland and seminal vesicles; also called seminal fluid.

Seminal vesicles: a pair of structures located near the urinary bladder and prostate gland that manufacture seminal fluid.

Sperm: the male reproductive cell, or sex cell.

Spermatic cord: a group of arteries, veins, lymph vessels, nerves, and the duct called the vas deferens that passes through the inguinal canal to the testes.

Testis: a testicle; the male gonad.

Uterus: the female womb.

Vagina: the female sex organ; also the birth canal.

Vulva: the visible external female genitalia, including the mons pubis, labia, clitoris, vaginal orifice, vestibule, and vestibular glands.

PATHOLOGY OF THE REPRODUCTIVE SYSTEM

The reproductive system is susceptible to the same pathologies that can affect the rest of the body, including viral, bacterial, or fungal infections, cancer, and birth defects. **Infertility** in either sex is a medical specialty unto itself. Medical technology has advanced to the stage that almost anyone can have a child through one means or another, regardless of their medical problems. For example, **surrogacy** is the use of another mother (a surrogate) to carry the fetus, which might have been created in a test tube using harvested eggs and donated sperm.

Sexually transmitted diseases include **AIDS, HIV infection, chlamydia, herpes, gonorrhea, syphilis,** and other conditions in which the usual manner of spreading is sexual contact. According to the Centers for Disease Control and Prevention (CDC), chlamydia is the most prevalent STD in the United States, with more than 850,000 cases reported in 2002, compared with 26,000 cases of AIDS reported in 2002. The actual number is probably much higher than reported for chlamydia (and all STDs) because many people, especially the poor, do not seek medical care and thus go unreported. If allowed to go untreated, chlamydia can lead to many other problems such as ectopic pregnancy and pelvic inflammatory disease (PID). Chlamydia is dangerous because infected women often experience no symptoms and unknowingly pass it on to their sexual partners. It can also be passed on to the baby during childbirth and can cause pneumonia and other complications in newborns.

A word about massage is in order here. You are not going to get AIDS by massaging someone who has it. If a person is in an advanced state and has active skin lesions caused by **Kaposi's** sarcoma, a form of cancer that often accompanies HIV/AIDS, you can avoid those areas and still give a massage. People are often wary of touching a person with AIDS, but there is no need to be. They need to be touched like the rest of the population, and in fact probably need it more. However, human papilloma virus (HPV) and herpes *can* be contracted by direct skin contact with an infected person, even if they do not have any obvious lesions. Caution is required; you may want to wear protective gloves or perform modalities during which the infected client remains clothed.

Abruptio placentae: premature separation of the placenta; life-threatening to the fetus.

AIDS (acquired immunodeficiency syndrome): a disease that is epidemic in prevalence, caused by the human immunodeficiency virus (HIV).

Amenorrhea: the (abnormal) discontinuation of the menstrual cycle. Primary amenorrhea is the condition of a woman having never menstruated; secondary amenorrhea is commonly seen in endurance athletes who have very low body fat, and in anorexics.

Bartholin cyst: a cyst in the vestibular gland.

Benign prostatic hypertrophy (BPH): a noncancerous enlargement of the prostate gland.

Body lice: small parasitic insects that cause a red rash; their eggs stick to hair shafts and cause itching.

Breast cancer: the uncontrolled growth of abnormal breast tissue.

Breast lump: a general term for any lump in the breast—tumor, cyst, or abscess; can be benign or malignant.

Candidiasis: a superficial fungal infection caused by *Candida albicans* that usually involves the skin, mucous membranes, respiratory tract, or vagina.

Castration: the removal or destruction of the testes.

Cervical cancer: cancer at the neck of the uterus.

Chlamydia: the most common bacterial sexually transmitted disease.

Chronic cervicitis: a lingering or recurrent inflammation of the cervix.

Circumcision: the surgical removal of the foreskin of the penis.

Cryptorchism: the failure of one or both of the testes to descend.

Dysmenorrhea: difficulty with menses accompanied by pain.

Ectopic pregnancy: the abnormal growth of the fetus somewhere other than the uterus, usually in the fallopian tubes.

Endometriosis: the abnormal growth of tissue resembling the lining of the uterus in places other than the uterus, including the fallopian tubes and pelvic cavity. Occurrence in the fallopian tubes is significant for risk for infertility.

Erectile dysfunction: the inability to maintain an erection for sexual intercourse.

Fibrocystic breast disease: a chronic disorder of forming abnormal fibrous tissue in the breasts.

Fibroid: a nonmalignant tumor of smooth muscle in the uterus.

Gardnerella (haemophilus) vaginitis: a bacterial inflammation of the vagina that usually occurs in children and in women who have not had any sexual contact.

Genital herpes: a sexually transmitted disease caused by a herpes virus, characterized by painful outbreaks of lesions on the external genitals.

Genital warts: warts that thrive on the moist skin of the sex organs, caused by the human papilloma virus (HPV).

Gonorrhea: a sexually transmitted disease caused by bacteria and characterized by pus discharge and painful urination.

Hepatitis B: a viral disease, spread by contact with contaminated blood or passed through the placenta from mother to child; a person can be a carrier and be asymptomatic; severe infections are characteristic, as is cirrhosis of the liver. Also called serum hepatitis.

Hermaphroditism: the condition of one individual having sex organs characteristic of both male and female.

Hypospadias: a birth defect in which the urethra opens at the bottom surface of the penis.

Hysterectomy: surgical removal of the uterus.

Impotence: the inability to obtain or maintain an erection.

Infertility: the inability to sexually reproduce.

Leukorrhea: a white, sticky discharge from the vagina.

Orchitis: an inflammation of a testicle.

Ovarian cancer: a malignant tumor of the ovary.

Pelvic inflammatory disease (PID): an inflammatory condition of the pelvic cavity that is secondary to another disease.

Phimosis: a condition in which the foreskin cannot be drawn back over the penis.

Placenta previa: a condition in which the placenta covers the opening to the birth canal.

Premenstrual syndrome (PMS): a combination of physical discomfort and mental and emotional upset that normally occurs between ovulation and the onset of menstruation.

Prostate cancer: a malignant tumor of the prostate gland.

Prostate disorder: any dysfunction affecting the prostate gland.

Prostatitis: an inflammation of the prostate gland.

Radical mastectomy: a total removal of the breast, surrounding tissue, and lymph nodes in response to breast cancer.

Salpingitis: an inflammation of the Fallopian tubes.

Syphilis: a serious sexually transmitted disease caused by a spirochete (a bacterium).

Testicular cancer: a malignancy of the testicles.

Toxic shock syndrome: a serious bloodborne bacterial infection that if allowed to progress can result in kidney failure or shock.

Trichomoniasis: an inflammation of the vagina caused by the protozoan *Trichomonas vaginitis.*

Uterine cancer: a malignancy of the uterus.

Uterine disorder: any malfunction of the uterus.

Vaginitis: an inflammation of the vagina usually accompanied by burning, itching, and foul-smelling discharge.

Yeast vaginitis: another term for candidiasis; a yeast infection.

Tips for Passing

If you are an auditory learner rather than a visual learner, read the definitions and other information into a small tape recorder, and listen to the tape at every opportunity.

I commuted to a school that was more than an hour's drive from my home. I would tape lectures and books I needed to read for classes and play them during the drive. It works! Look at how much time most people waste during a day while waiting at the doctor's office, waiting in line, etc. Take advantage of that time to study, whether listening to a tape or reading a book. Try playing the tape when you go to bed and listen to it as you are falling asleep. Listen to the tape while you walk or work out.

Affirmation

I apply my best effort to the things that are important to me.

Practice Questions

1. Gonads refer to
   a. Ovaries
   b. Testes
   c. Both
   d. Neither

2. A chromosome that is not a sex chromosome is called a(n)
   a. Genosome
   b. Biosome
   c. Transome
   d. Autosome

3. Examples of secondary sex characteristics include the
   a. Vagina
   b. Breasts
   c. Uterus
   d. None of the above

4. The most common bacterial sexually transmitted disease is
   a. Syphilis
   b. AIDS
   c. Herpes
   d. Chlamydia

5. Genital herpes is caused by
   a. Bacteria
   b. Fungi
   c. Parasites
   d. Viruses

6. The abnormal growth of the fetus somewhere other than the uterus is called a(n)
   a. Ectopic pregnancy
   b. Myopic pregnancy
   c. Endopic pregnancy
   d. Toxemic pregnancy

7. The pair of structures near the prostate gland that manufacture semen are the
    a. Kidneys
    b. Seminal vesicles
    c. Ureters
    d. Lymph vessels

8. Gametes are produced by
    a. The ovaries
    b. The testes
    c. Both
    d. Neither

9. A cell containing all the genetic material is referred to as
    a. Diploid
    b. Haploid
    c. Endoid
    d. None of these

10. The onset of menstruation is
    a. Menopause
    b. Dysmenorrhea
    c. Menarche
    d. Amenorrhea

PART 3

Biomechanics and Kinesiology

CHAPTER 20

Safe and Efficient Movement for Client and Therapist

Knowledge is of two kinds. We know a subject ourselves, or we know where we can find information upon it.

—SAMUEL JOHNSON

HIGHLIGHTS

Biomechanics, sometimes referred to as **body mechanics,** is the mechanics of muscular activity in movement and exercise. **Kinesiology** is the study of the way the body moves and the body parts involved in any movement.

Kinesiology is divided into a number of subdisciplines. **Applied kinesiology** is a muscle testing modality developed in the 1960s by an American chiropractor, Dr. George Goodheart, as an evaluation tool for muscle function. **Specialized kinesiology,** sometimes referred to as **energy kinesiology,** also uses muscle testing and is a part of many modalities of body/mind therapy, including One Brain, Touch for Health, and Applied Neurogenics. The primary difference in the subdisciplines is that specialized kinesiology uses straight-armed muscle testing and involves verbal questions that can be answered "yes" or "no." Applied kinesiology uses hundreds of muscle tests but does not involve any verbal questioning. Applied kinesiology focuses on structure and function, whereas specialized kinesiology has a big focus on the emotional and energetic aspects of the client.

The massage therapist must be concerned with biomechanics and kinesiology on two levels. First, many clients may have pain from poor posture, restricted movement, or **repetitive motion injuries** (Fig. 20.1). Second, if the therapist does not move in a safe and efficient manner herself, she risks career-shortening injuries.

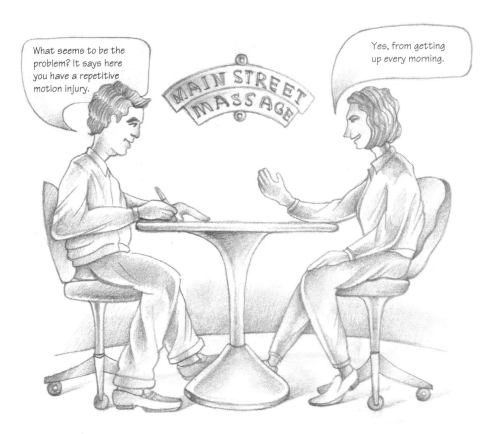

FIGURE 20.1
Repetitive motion injuries.

In American higher education, kinesiology is a respected field concerned with the science of movement that crosses into many other areas of study. Knowledge, methods of inquiry, and principles from traditional areas of study in the arts, humanities, and sciences are applied to such disciplines as exercise and sports physiology, biomechanics, biochemistry, molecular physiology, psychology, sports medicine, and ergonomics.

Ergonomics

Ergonomics is the application of scientific information to the needs of people in the design of objects, systems, and environments for human use. The term ergonomics is derived from two Greek words: *ergon* meaning "work" and *nomo* meaning "by natural laws." Ergonomics incorporates information from anatomy, physiology, kinesiology, psychology, and design to optimize human performance while recognizing limitations and safety concerns. Take a walk through your workspace with an eye toward recognizing potential ergonomic concerns: the height of items, adequate lighting, sharp corners sticking out, and things placed where they are most accessible without your having to twist or bend.

Look through your client's eyes, also. Clients come in different shapes and sizes and include the elderly and the handicapped. Does your workspace accommodate everyone with ease? A word of advice: An upstairs office is not a good idea, unless your building has an elevator. A staircase leaves out wheelchair-bound clients, and people with sciatic pain don't want to climb a flight of stairs. Older clients or those with arthritis may seek a massage therapist with an office that is more easily accessible.

The following basic principles govern the discipline of ergonomics:

1. All work activities should allow the worker to assume several different, but equally healthy and safe, postures.

2. When muscular force has to be exerted, it should be exerted by the largest appropriate muscle groups available.

3. Work activities should be performed with the joints at about the midpoint of their range of motion. This applies particularly to the head, neck, and upper limbs.

Performing massage can be strenuous, especially if you are working in a setting in which you may be seeing many clients per day. Being aware of your biomechanics and the ergonomics in your workspace will ultimately extend your career for many years.

Taking Care of Yourself

As therapists, we create our own problems by working on a table that is the incorrect height, bending at the waist, and applying all our pressure with our thumbs. If you are working in an office and spending time at the computer or otherwise sitting at a desk, that's a consideration as well. Getting up and taking frequent stretching breaks is a simple thing that can make a big difference in the way you feel at the end of the workday. The best scenario is a workday in which you can alternate between sitting and standing. When performing massage, I usually sit while working on the head and feet, and stand while working on the rest of the body. I even get some exercise, when the client is prone, by doing a few stretches of my own. Depending on the type of floor that is in your workspace, you may want to get a thick carpet or rubber fatigue mat to place under your table and in the surrounding floor space where you are standing.

In the office area, you can't usually adjust the height of your desk, but you can get an adjustable chair, a separate keyboard shelf, and gel pads for wrist support. A footrest and an adjustable monitor stand are also worthwhile investments. On days when you are taking care of administrative details or writing, stand and stretch after every page or two. A good office chair is one that has lumbar support. If your chair does not fit that description, either buy a new one or at least get a lumbar pillow. It should support the small of your back. A lumbar pillow is also a good idea in the car if your seat doesn't adjust to suit you. The ideal seat has a clearance between the back of your knees and the edge of your seat. Otherwise the chair tends to cut right across the sciatic nerve and causes the pain, stiffness, or numbness known as **sciatica.** Your knees should be at approximately the same height as your hips to avoid putting undue pressure on the legs or gluteals. The armrests should be at the correct height to loosely support the arms near the torso. Positioning the keyboard and mouse so that your wrists are straight in a **neutral position** can keep you from getting **carpal tunnel syndrome.**

The use of proper biomechanics increases the length of a therapist's career by decreasing the possibility of injury. It improves the strength and effectiveness of the massage, keeps the therapist from getting tired, and enhances the client's experience. The therapist should be moving smoothly and efficiently. Proper biomechanics were addressed during the first day of class at the massage school I attended, and that should be the case in every school. Poor habits once established are hard to break, so it is best to start with proper movement patterns from the very first massage. The table should be at your most comfortable height for working, and it may need to be changed to accommodate different sizes of clients. Keep your back straight and your knees slightly bent. Let your lower body—not just your hands—provide the pressure. Work from the center of your pelvis, and allow your legs to do most of the work. Keep elbows close to the body and wrists relaxed. Make use of your forearms and elbows for pressure work or deep, gliding strokes. Above all, be conscious of your body and your movement. If a particular movement is causing you discomfort, make the necessary adjustment in your posture or technique. For example, I like using Shiatsu, but my knees suffer when I do it on the floor, so I lower my table to the lowest setting and that way I still have leverage but I'm not uncomfortable. In the unfortunate event that you do have an injury, follow the same advice you would give a client: Let it rest so it has time to heal. Using proper biomechanics will keep you energized and efficient throughout the day.

Finally, take care of your own hands. They are your livelihood. **Hyperextensions,** such as hyperextending a thumb, is painful. Work smart, not hard. Right now you are just starting out, and you may think it's cool to massage for 10 hours straight and go home with more money in a day than you used to make in a week. That's not a wise idea. If you want to still be doing massage 10 years from now, pace yourself and take care of yourself. Some therapists burn out 2 years after graduation by trying to do too much and injuring themselves. Vary your routine.

Taking Care of the Client

Many of the problems we see in massage practices, such as carpal tunnel syndrome and sciatica, can be improved (along with massage) by simple changes in habits. It is up to you—the therapist—to educate the client about such things. A case in point is men who carry a wallet in their back pockets; this "hip hike" is a recipe for sciatic pain. (I give all my male clients a warning about the wallet in the pocket.) Schoolchildren who carry heavy book bags are likely to have biomechanical problems. Women who carry heavy shoulder bags or always carry their toddler on one hip are obvious examples of clients who are physically out of balance.

Sharing simple office tips and stretching exercises with your clients is part of your obligation to educate those with whom you work. Use your intake form to ask people what kind of work they do and what kind of activities they participate in. This will give you some insight into why their body is in the shape it's in and what stretches or modifications you can tell them about to help their particular situation.

The Body in Balance

Balance has been described as the ability of an individual to maintain his or her body's **center of gravity** over the base of support, whether that base of support is stationary, **static balance,** or moving, **dynamic balance.** While maintaining balance, a person responds to both external forces that can destabilize the body's center of gravity and internal forces that result from the body's movements. Understanding biomechanics is understanding how the body comes out of balance and how you as a therapist can work to restore that balance. Three systems are involved in the body's structural balance: the visual system, the vestibular system, and the somatosensory system.

The **visual system** is constantly giving us cues: lean forward to walk up that hill; step sideways to avoid that obstacle. Cues about position and depth perception aid our every movement.

Proprioception is the ongoing process of self-regulation of the movements and posture of the body through the **somatosensory system,** beginning with stimuli from the receptors in the musculoskeletal system. The **vestibular system** of the inner ear, or labyrinth, also has receptors that help govern our balance. Proprioceptors provide us with sensations that let us know how a muscle or tendon is contracted and how a movement is taking place relative to the joints and muscles. Proprioception allows us to move without thinking about it. The main structures involved in proprioception are the **joints, muscles,** and **tendons.**

Afferent signals sent to the central nervous system by the three sensory systems are processed at the spinal cord (reflex activations), the lower brain and midbrain (automatic activations), and the cerebral cortex (voluntary movements). The processing of sensory information at each of these levels is vital to maintaining the body's balance. Once information is received and processed, a response is executed by the muscular system to maintain balance. If any of the systems is impaired, the body's ability to maintain postural balance is challenged.

The English physicist Sir Isaac Newton identified three laws of motion:

1. Every body continues in a state of rest, or uniform motion, in a line, unless it is compelled to change that state by forces impressed on it.

2. The change of motion is proportional to the force applied and made in the direction in which that force is impressed.

3. To every action there is always an opposite and equal reaction; or the mutual actions of two bodies on each other are always equal and directed to the contrary parts.

In the body, there are three components that illustrate these principles. The **agonist** is the main muscle that initiates any particular motion. The **synergist** is a muscle or muscles that help the agonist perform a particular motion. The **antagonist** is a muscle that works *against* another muscle or performs an opposing motion.

Levers are discussed in Chapter 8 on the skeletal system, but here's a quick review. For movement to occur, bones act as **levers.** The joints function as the **fulcrums** of these levers. Three factors affect how much a bone is going to move: the position of the fulcrum (joint), the effort required to move, and the resistance encountered. Levers are classified into three different types, according to these three factors. **First-class levers,** the most rare in the human body, can be a mechanical advantage or disadvantage, depending on whether the fulcrum is close to the resistance. The best example is the head as it rests on the vertebral column. In a **second-class lever,** the resistance is between the fulcrum (joint) and the effort. Second-class levers are not plentiful in the human body, either. One example is the ball of the foot, combined with the tarsals and the calf muscles. The most plentiful levers in the body are **third-class levers,** which include the elbow joint and the adductors of the thighs.

WHAT YOU NEED TO KNOW

Applied kinesiology: a system of muscle testing used to assess neuromuscular function as it relates to structural, chemical, and mental functioning.

Biomechanical: referring to a mechanical analysis of body motion.

Ergonomics: the study of human factors in the context of the work environment.

Kinesthesia: the sensory perception of muscle movement.

Neutral position: neither flexed nor extended; basically straight.

Perception: the conscious awareness of a stimulus.

Receptor: the sensory nerve ending that responds to a stimulus.

Sensation: a change in consciousness that may be brought about by an external stimulus or an internal change in the body.

PATHOLOGY RELATED TO BIOMECHANICS

Pathological conditions related to biomechanics can take various forms. Many birth defects, diseases, and injuries can interfere with the body's ability to move and function normally. A simple strain or sprain is enough to interfere with movement. Many pathologies of the central nervous system cause deterioration and, sometimes, permanent loss of normal movement. Spinal cord injuries often cause serious instantaneous permanent loss of movement. The normal aging process tends to slow our movements. Unfortunately, diseases such as rheumatoid arthritis are not limited to the elderly and can cause loss of movement in young people. Many conditions affecting movement can be improved through massage and physical therapy. Even people with permanent loss of movement gain circulatory benefits from massage.

 Tips for Passing

You can only avoid procrastinating by getting down to the business at hand: preparing to take the examination. If you have lost sight of your goals, have a serious talk with yourself. Remind yourself why you have invested time and money in going to school. Discipline gets easier each time you practice it, and the payoff is passing the test.

Affirmation

I am truly looking forward to passing the examination.

Practice Questions

1. Another term for the inner ear is the
   a. Reticulum
   b. Arachnoid
   c. Labyrinth
   d. Copia

2. The main muscle responsible for any movement is the
   a. Synergist
   b. Antagonist
   c. Protagonist
   d. Agonist

3. _____ allows us to move without thinking about it.
   a. Proprioception
   b. Stimulus
   c. Flexion
   d. Extension

4. Ergonomics is concerned with _____ factors pertaining to the environment.
   a. Mineral
   b. Animal

    c. Human

    d. Vegetable

5. The three laws of motion were identified by
   a. Sir Isaac Newton
   b. Sir Stephen Newton
   c. Dr. Stephen Hawking
   d. Galileo

6. The factors that affect how or how much a bone is going to move are the
   a. Position of the joint
   b. Resistance encountered
   c. Effort required
   d. All of the above

7. The most rare lever in the body is the
   a. Second class lever
   b. Third class lever
   c. Fourth class lever
   d. None of these levers

8. Improper biomechanics can cause
   a. Injury
   b. Poor posture
   c. Carpal tunnel syndrome
   d. All of the above

9. The sensory perception of muscle movement is
   a. Myasthenia
   b. Kinesiology
   c. Kinesthesia
   d. Myasthology

10. An example of a second-class lever in the body is the
    a. Hip joint
    b. Elbow joint
    c. Atlas
    d. Ball of the foot

PART 4

Traditional Eastern Medicine

CHAPTER 21

Eastern Methods

The surest test of discipline is its absence.

—CLARA BARTON

HIGHLIGHTS

Traditional Eastern medicine is a combination of anatomy, physiology, pathology, and philosophy. The Chinese, as well as other Asians and Eastern peoples, have practiced holistic medicine for centuries. Many forms of bodywork have their basis in Eastern philosophy: **shiatsu, acupuncture/acupressure, Usui Reiki,** and **amma** (sometimes referred to as **anma**), to name just a few. **Touch for Health** is based on the meridians, although it is not an Eastern method. **Meridians** can be thought of as energy pathways in the body. (A more thorough explanation of the meridians is given in Chapter 22.) The universal theme among these traditions is the concept of **chi, ki,** or **qi**—the idea of a **life force** or **bioenergy** (Fig. 21.1).

At the basis of Oriental medicine is also the theory of **yin and yang,** which represents the opposing principles of the universe. **Yin** represents the principles of femaleness, the moon, completion, cold, darkness, material forms, and submission. **Yang** represents the principles of maleness, the sun, creation, heat, light, and dominance. Each of these opposites produces the other: heaven creates the ideas of things under yang, the earth produces their material forms under yin, and vice versa; creation occurs under the principle of yang, the completion of the created thing occurs under yin, and vice versa; and so on. This production of yin from yang and yang from yin occurs cyclically and constantly, so that no one principle continually dominates the other or determines the other. All opposites that one experiences—health and illness, abundance and poverty, power and submission—can be explained in reference to the temporary dominance of one principle over the other. Neither principle dominates perpetu-

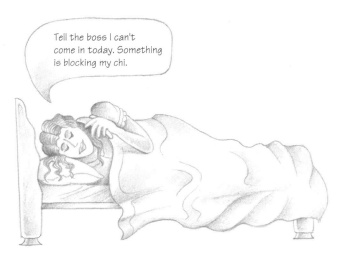

FIGURE 21.1
Blocked chi.

ally. All conditions are subject to change into their opposites. Yin flows up from the earth, whereas yang flows down from the sun.

Yin and yang are also tied to the theory of **wu-hsing,** or the **Five Elements.** These five material agents are **wood, fire, earth, metal,** and **water.** They are grouped either in the order by which they produce one another: wood gives rise to fire, fire gives rise to earth, earth gives rise to metal, metal gives rise to water, water gives rise to wood; or in the order by which they are conquered by one another: fire is conquered by water, water is conquered by earth, earth is conquered by wood, wood is conquered by metal, and metal is conquered by fire, and so on. Each of these sequences can be used to explain the progression of change in the body and in the universe and to illustrate that all things exist always; they just change form.

Anatomically, the upper part of the body, the exterior part of the body, and the back are all yang. The lower part of the body, the interior part of the body, and the abdomen are all yin. Each organ has some properties that are yin and some that are yang. In Eastern pathology, diseases that present with heat symptoms are usually yang, whereas diseases that present with cold symptoms are usually yin.

In traditional Eastern medicine, blood is viewed as the body's manifestation of energy. The spleen and stomach are considered the main sources of qi and blood because they are considered the starting point of the transformational process that turns our food and water intake into blood. After the stomach receives the food, the spleen extracts the qi from the food and sends it to the lungs, where it mixes with the qi from the air and is then sent to the heart to be mixed with the body's primary qi to produce blood. Blood then travels throughout the body to nourish the organs and tissues, and it is also regarded as the origin of mental faculties.

Some students may object to the concepts of Oriental medicine. However, the NCE includes questions about Eastern methods, so you need to be prepared.

Many Eastern methods of health care and bodywork are in popular use in the United States and all over the world. A quick Internet search identifies more than 100 schools of Oriental medicine in the US alone.

There are many different types of Oriental bodywork. **Tui Na,** like all the other forms of Oriental bodywork, is distinctly different from Western types of massage because Eastern modalities are based on the energetic framework of the body, much like acupuncture and herbology. Western methods are mainly directed at the musculoskeletal system, although some practitioners work from a body/mind/spirit standpoint. Although the goal of Swedish massage is to relax tense muscles, Oriental bodywork attempts to influence the energetic facets of the same tense muscles, usually by applying pressure techniques. Tui Na is distinct from other types of Oriental bodywork (such as shiatsu) because of the nature of the techniques used to influence the energetic framework; many of the Tui Na techniques involve sophisticated hand movements and are not dependent only on pressure techniques.

Chi Nei Tsang (CNT) means "working the energy of the internal organs" or "internal organs chi transformation." This modality uses the principles of Kung Fu and Tai Chi Chuan, known as **Chi-Kung.** CNT practitioners are trained in Chi-Kung and work mainly on the abdomen with deep, gentle touch to train the internal organs to work more efficiently and to help process unresolved emotional issues. All the body systems are addressed: digestive, respiratory, lymphatic, nervous, endocrine, urinary, reproductive, muscular, and skeletal, as well as the meridians.

Another modality with many different forms is **shiatsu.** Instead of strictly working on the meridians, shiatsu addresses points called **tsubos** with applied acupressure to release blockages. Shiatsu and other Oriental modalities are often performed on mats on the floor with the client fully clothed. In the practice of Oriental bodywork, the cun is used as a measurement from one point to another. A **cun** is basically an anatomical inch, equal to the distance from the distal crease to the middle crease of the finger (of the client, not the practitioner).

Ayurveda, or **Ayurvedic medicine,** from India, has much in common with Oriental medicine, although the terminology is different. Energy is called **prana** or **Kundalini.** In Ayurveda, energy points are referred to as **marmas.** Ayurveda is at least 5000 years old. Like Chinese medicine, Ayurveda is a "complete science of life." Proper breathing, nutrition, and exercise are all required to keep the body in balance. This ancient Indian philosophy of health and healing, based on food, lifestyle, and one's individual constitutional makeup, follows the principle that we are all made up of the five elements of ether (space), air, fire, water, and earth, and that these elements in different combinations are responsible for physiological functions, called **doshas,** or humors. Note that these five elements differ from wu-hsing theory. Each person is made up of a unique combination of all the doshas, but one dosha is usually dominant over the others.

There are three types of doshas: the vata, the pitta, and the kapha. Ether and air combine to form **vata dosha.** Vata governs the principle of movement. It therefore can be seen as the force that directs nerve impulses, circulation, respiration, and elimination. Vata is dry, cold, and light and corresponds to the element air. Fire and water are the elements that combine to form **pitta dosha,** the process of transformation or metabolism. The transformation of foods into nutrients that our body can assimilate is an example of a pitta function. Pitta is also responsible for metabolism in the organ and tissue systems, as well as cellular metabolism. Pitta is oily, hot, and light and corresponds to the element fire. Water and earth elements combine to form the **kapha dosha,** which is responsible for growth, adding structure unit by unit. Another function of the kapha dosha is to offer protection. Cerebrospinal fluid protects the brain and spinal column and is a type of kapha found in the body. The mucous lining of the stomach is another example of the kapha dosha protecting the tissues. Kapha is wet, cold, and heavy and corresponds to the element water.

Cleansing the body from an Ayurvedic standpoint means to rid oneself not only of physical ills but also of mental and spiritual ills. It is interesting to note that the exercises practiced by Asians and other Easterners are gentle and graceful exercises, such as T'ai Chi and yoga, not aerobic bouncing around or running on a treadmill, and yet obesity is not the problem in the East that it is in the West, and life expectancies are long. The traditional Eastern diet is also naturally low in fat.

WHAT YOU NEED TO KNOW

Acupressure: the application of pressure with the thumbs, fingers, or mechanical objects into living tissues for remedial purposes; follows the principles of acupuncture in Oriental medicine, performed along specific places on the meridians to release energy blockages. Also used generally as a term for specific pressure.

Acupuncture: the insertion of fine needles into living tissues for remedial purposes; in Oriental medicine, performed along specific places on the meridians to release energy blockages.

Amma: traditional Asian massage. Using no oil, amma involves stretching, squeezing, and massaging to stimulate the body to become and/or remain healthy. Amma focuses on improving muscle condition and the circulation of ki, or universal life energy. Also referred to as anma.

Brahmand: the cosmos, the universe.

Cun: a measurement used in acupuncture, the distance between the distal crease and the middle crease of the finger of the client.

Dharma: a term with no literal English translation, whose approximate meaning is "natural law," or those principles of reality that are the very nature and design of the universe.

Hara: the lower belly just under the navel, the "vital center" of physical and mental stability.

Jitsu: having excessive energy.

Kata: a Japanese term meaning mold, model, style, shape, or form.

Kundalini: the cosmic energy believed to be present in everyone.

Kyo: lacking in energy.

Marma: a pressure point in Ayurvedic massage; many marmas correspond to acupuncture or shiatsu points.

Moxibustion: in traditional Chinese medicine, a technique to stimulate and strengthen the blood and the life energy, or qi, of the body. A stick or cone of burning mug wort, *Artemisia vulgaris,* is placed over an inflamed or affected area on the body; the cone is placed on an acupuncture point and burned. The cone is removed before burning the skin.

Nadi: an Indian term for meridian, meaning "river."

Prana: a Sanskrit word meaning "life force," bioenergy, or vital energy that keeps the body alive and maintains a state of good health.

Shiatsu: a Japanese method of bodywork performed on the floor; acupressure is applied along a series of points (tsubos) to release blocked energy.

Srota: in Ayurvedic medicine, a body passage or channel that carries solids, liquids, gases, nerve impulses, nutrients, waste products, and/or secretions.

Sushumna: in Ayurvedic medicine, the main meridian (nadi) that runs up the center of the spine.

Tao: a Japanese word (pronounced "dow"), roughly translated as "path," or "the way." Tao is a power that surrounds and flows through all things, living and nonliving. It is the regulator of natural processes and nourishes balance in the universe. Tao embodies the harmony of opposites (light/dark, male/female, yin/yang).

 ## Tips for Passing

Make an agreement with yourself, such as "no television until I have studied for an hour," and stick to it. If you have school-age children, sit down and study with them while they are doing their homework. They'll think it's cool that mom or dad has to do homework, too, and it may even save some of the whining that goes on about it! Plus, it's quality time with your children.

Practice Questions

1. Yin and yang represent
   a. Two extraordinary meridians
   b. The main religion of China
   c. The opposite principles of the universe
   d. A type of Oriental bodywork

2. The Sanskrit word that means "life force" is
   a. Kata
   b. Prana
   c. Karma
   d. Vata

3. The hara is located
   a. In the pineal gland
   b. Above the heart
   c. Just below the navel
   d. At the perineum

4. The path that is followed by sushumna goes
   a. Up the center of the spine
   b. Down the sciatic nerve
   c. Through the digestive tract
   d. Down the windpipe

5. For clients who need to do gentle stretching exercises at home, you might suggest
   a. Tae Kwan Do
   b. Tui Na
   c. Reiki
   d. Tai Chi

6. The dosha that is described as wet, cold, and heavy corresponds to the element water is called
   a. Vata
   b. Kapha
   c. Pitta
   d. Prana

Affirmation

My strength is my determination.

7. Nadis and srotas are both
   a. Channels
   b. Bony prominences
   c. Another term for the sex organs
   d. A form of Japanese bodywork

8. Wu-hsing is the Chinese term for
   a. Kundalini
   b. Ayurveda
   c. The Five Elements
   d. A form of Japanese bodywork

9. To state that a point on the body is jitsu means that it is
   a. An area that is infected
   b. An area that is lacking in energy
   c. An area that has too much energy
   d. An area that is numb

10. In Ayurvedic massage, energy points are referred to as
    a. Trigger points
    b. Dharmas
    c. Karmas
    d. Marmas

CHAPTER 22

The Meridians

The cure for sorrow is to learn something.

—Barbara Sher

HIGHLIGHTS

When I first heard the term **meridian,** it was a foreign concept. I understood that the brain needs electricity to work, that the heart needs electricity to beat, and the neurons need electricity to fire. It stands to reason that the electricity in the body is organized in some way, not just randomly, and this is the basis of meridian theory: The body has **energy pathways.** There are differences in meridian theory between the cultures of the Chinese and the Japanese. The meridians are shown in Figure 22.1. In the figure, notice that anatomical position in Chinese theory is different from anatomical position in Western theory; the arms are extended at shoulder height and bent at the elbow in the traditional Chinese way.

It is advisable for massage therapists to know the meridians—their organ associations, the major treatment points located along each meridian, and their major characteristics, particularly where they begin and end. As it would be impossible to list even 10% of the treatment points here, you'll want to study a more complete text or chart.

Here are some of the more important treatment points. LI 4, located on the back of the hand in the web between the thumb and the index finger, is often referred to as "the great eliminator" because stimulating that point can relieve constipation as well as the headache that often accompanies that condition. K 27 is in the depression on the lower border of the clavicle and can be self-stimulated when you need energy. GV 26 is slightly above the middle of the philtrum, the area under the nose. Stimulation of GV 26 relieves back pain and calms nervous system disorders. SP 6 is located directly above the medial malleolus; this and many other points are to be avoided on pregnant women because stimulation can cause uterine contractions.

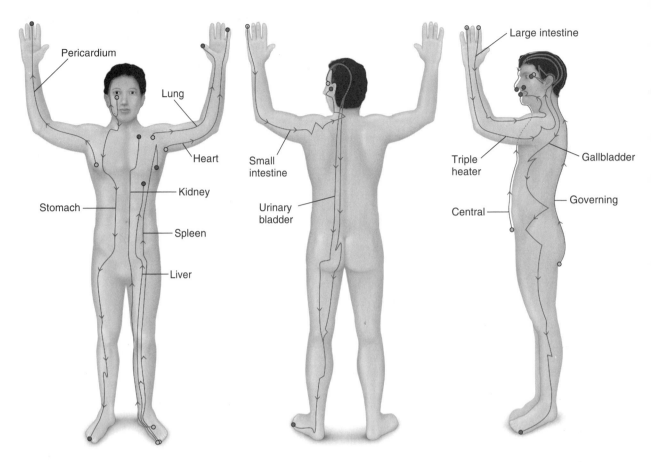

FIGURE 22.1
The meridians: the body's energy pathways. (Reprinted with permission from Braun MB, Simonson S. Introduction to Massage Therapy. Baltimore: Lippincott Williams & Wilkins, 2005:440. Fig. 13-5.)

There are 12 primary meridians and two extraordinary meridians. The 12 **primary meridians** run in pairs, one along either side of the body, mirroring the other. The heart governor (HG) is paired with the triple warmer (TW), the heart (HT) meridian is paired with the small intestine (SI) meridian, the urinary bladder (UB) is paired with the kidney (K), the stomach (ST) is paired with the spleen (SP), the gallbladder (GB) is paired with the liver (LV), and the lung (LU) is paired with the large intestine (LI) meridian. The two **extraordinary meridians,** called the conception vessel (CV) and the governing vessel (GV), run around the torso and are not paired.

The earliest known book about meridian theory was published more than 2,000 years ago, and the first on **acupuncture,** the medical art of using fine needles to stimulate points along the meridians, was published in the early 1500s. Current Chinese theory holds that at least 500 important meridian points have been identified and that still more remain to be discovered. Simply stated, the theory is that a blockage in the meridian can cause disease in the body, and that by releasing the blockage, the normal flow of energy—and thus good health—can be restored. Some modalities, such as shiatsu, use finger pressure called **acupressure,** instead of needles, to stimulate meridian points.

In Chinese medicine, meridian theory believes that the body's chi circulates through each organ in a 12-hour period, and each organ has an associated time when the energy peaks in that particular organ. In Chinese medicine, however, the organs

TABLE 22.1   The Meridians and Their Characteristics

Meridian and How It Is Paired	Location	Associated Element	Yin/ Yang	Associated Color	Associated Season and Time
Lung (LU); paired with large intestine (LI)	Begins at chest, up arm, ends at thumb	Metal	Yin	White	Autumn 3 am
Large intestine (LI); paired with lung	Begins at index finger, up arm and neck, ends at nose	Metal	Yang	White	Autumn 5 am
Stomach (S); paired with spleen (SP)	Begins at eye, down anterior body, ends at second toe	Earth	Yang	Yellow	Late summer 7am
Spleen (SP); paired with stomach (ST)	Begins at big toe, up inside of leg, up anterior body, ends at underarm	Earth	Yin	Yellow	Late summer 9am
Heart (HT); paired with small intestine (SI)	Begins at underarm, up medial arm, ends at little finger	Fire	Yin	Red	Summer 11am
Small intestine (SI); paired with heart	Begins at little finger, down lateral arm, up the neck, ends in front of ear	Fire	Yang	Red	Summer 1 pm
Urinary bladder (UB), also referred to as bladder (BL); paired with kidney (K)	Begins at eye, over head down back and posterior leg, ends at little toe	Water	Yang	Black	Winter 3 pm
Kidney (K); paired with urinary bladder (UB)	Begins on bottom of foot, up medial leg and torso, ends at chest	Water	Yin	Black	Winter 5 pm
Circulation sex, also referred to as pericardium, heart governor (HG), heart protector, heart envelope, or heart constrictor	Begins at lateral chest, up medial arms, ends at middle finger	Fire	Yin	None	Summer 7 pm
Triple warmer (TW), also referred to as triple heater, triple burner, triple energizer, three burning spaces, or San Jiao; not paired	Begins at fourth finger, up posterior arm and lateral neck, ends on lateral head	Fire	Yang	None	Summer 9 pm
Gallbladder (GB)	Begins on lateral head, down lateral side of body, ends at fourth toe	Wood	Yang	Green	Spring 11 pm
Liver (LV or Li); paired with gallbladder (GB)	Begins on big toe, up medial leg, ends at 6th intercostal space	Wood	Yin	Green	Spring 1 am
Central (CV); also called conception vessel; not paired	Begins at perineum, up midsagittal line of torso, ends at mentolabial groove between chin and lower lip	None	Yin	None	None
Governing vessel (GV); not paired	Begins at coccyx, up midsagittal line of back and over head, ends at upper lip	None	Yang	None	None

are not strictly the same as in Western medicine. For instance, the kidney (K) meridian governs the adrenal glands and endocrine system; the urinary bladder (UB) meridian governs the kidneys and the urinary system. The meridians have many associations: organs, seasons, times of day, colors, emotions, elements, smells, directions, and so on. There are five seasons recognized in Chinese medicine; late summer is counted as a separate season and is noted as a time of change. The meridians and some of their associations are listed in Table 22.1.

If you have not performed and/or received any Eastern modalities of bodywork from a trained professional, make an appointment with a practitioner. You may find the work too relaxing to ask too many questions, but most practitioners will be glad to explain if you express interest.

WHAT YOU NEED TO KNOW

Instead of a list of definitions, Table 22.1 should help you learn what you need to know about the meridians.

 Tips for Passing

Ask a fellow student to trace the meridians on your body, and then reverse roles. Once is not enough!

Practice Questions

1. The term meridian is used to describe a(an)
   a. Nerve plexus
   b. Energy blockage
   c. Energy pathway
   d. None of the above

2. All together, there are _____ primary meridians.
   a. 10
   b. 12
   c. 14
   d. 16

3. The conception vessel and governing vessel are referred to as _____ meridians.
   a. Extraordinary
   b. Unnecessary
   c. Sudiferous
   d. Minor

4. Which of the following meridians is not associated with Yang?
   a. Large intestine (LI)
   b. Small intestine (SI)
   c. Liver (LV)
   d. Stomach (ST)

Affirmation

My chi flows effortlessly. I have all the energy I need.

5. In Chinese medicine theory, what circulates through the organs every 12 hours?
   a. Blood
   b. Hormones
   c. Chi
   d. Fresh oxygen

6. The two meridians that do not have any element associated with them are the
   a. Central and lung
   b. Lung and liver
   c. Circulation sex and governing
   d. Central and governing

7. The central meridian is also referred to as the
   a. Heart meridian
   b. Conception vessel
   c. Heart governor
   d. Circulation sex

8. The meridians that do not occur in pairs are the
   a. Central and governing
   b. Triple warmer
   c. Lung and kidney
   d. None of the above

9. The heart governor meridian is paired with the _____ meridian.
   a. Kidney
   b. Spleen
   c. Triple warmer
   d. Small intestine

10. The meridians that do not have an association with the elements are the
    a. Ordinary meridians
    b. Extraordinary meridians
    c. Stomach and spleen meridians
    d. Kidney and bladder meridians

CHAPTER 23

The Chakras

The beginning of knowledge is the discovery of something we do not understand.

—FRANK HERBERT

HIGHLIGHTS

Chakra is a Sanskrit word from ancient India meaning "wheel" or "disk." At the inner core of each one of us spin seven wheel-like energy centers, or chakras, which together form a system. There are also many minor chakras. Chakras are sites within the body that project as patterns of electromagnetic activity focused around the seven major spinal nerve ganglia and plexuses. They can be compared with valves, regulating the energy within our system, just as valves help regulate the flow of blood in the circulatory system. Each of the chakras is associated with an endocrine gland. The seven primary chakras are a kind of vortex or gathering point of organized life energy. Their interactions with the physical body occur through the endocrine glands and through the central nervous system. The chakras are affected by stress and emotional states. Fear, grief, anxiety, and other negative emotions directly affect chakra balance (and thus the endocrine and nervous systems).

In brief, the chakras have specific associations to locations of the body, colors, glands, body parts, emotions, and levels of consciousness. They are sometimes called the subtle body or the essential body. The chakras are also referred to by number; the crown is the seventh chakra and the numbers descend (Fig. 23.1).

Table 23.1 lists the chakras and their associations. As you review the associations, touch the chakra area. Visualize your chakras spinning in a steady, perfect, clockwise way as you touch each area. Visualize the color related to each chakra as you focus your attention on that area. Say it out loud. Visualize that the glands associated with

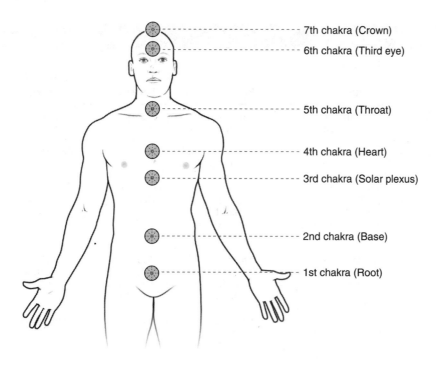

7th chakra (Crown)
6th chakra (Third eye)
5th chakra (Throat)
4th chakra (Heart)
3rd chakra (Solar plexus)
2nd chakra (Base)
1st chakra (Root)

FIGURE 23.1
The seven chakras.

each specific chakra are at optimum performance, carrying on the body's activities with perfect timing. Name it out loud. Have the intention that the emotions related to each chakra are in balance and serving you in the best way. Say them out loud, taking what is needed and releasing the rest. Listed are seven affirmations that correspond to the chakras. Say them out loud as you touch each chakra and visualize the associations of each chakra.

- At the crown: "I think positive thoughts."
- At the third eye: "I see the positive in everything."
- At the throat: "I speak only positive words."
- At the heart: "I feel positive with all my heart."
- At the solar plexus: "I manifest positive from the center of my being."
- At the base chakra: "My creations are all positive."
- At the root chakra: "My desires are positive."

There, you just gave yourself a chakra balance. Now commit to doing this simple process every day as you prepare for your examination—always out loud. This will reinforce your memory when you need it. Another method of chakra balancing is the color balance. You can do this by simply meditating on the color of the chakra that needs healing, using colored lights, or even wearing the colors associated with the chakras.

WHAT YOU NEED TO KNOW

Instead of a list of definitions, Table 23.1 should help you learn what you need to know about the chakras.

TABLE 23.1   The Chakras and Their Associations

Number	Name	Location	Color	Organs/ Body Parts	Gland/ Plexus	Senses	Emotions/ Area of Consciousness
Seventh chakra	Crown chakra	Top of head	Violet	Brain, nervous system	Pineal gland, limbic area		Empathy, unity separation
Sixth chakra	Third eye chakra	Center of forehead	Indigo	Forehead, temples	Pituitary gland, carotid plexus		Perception, spirituality
Fifth chakra	Throat chakra	Base of throat	Sky blue	Throat, neck, upper extremities	Thyroid gland, branchial plexus	Hearing	Expression, communication, creativity
Fourth chakra	Heart chakra	Center of chest	Emerald green	Heart, circulatory system, lungs, chest	Thymus gland, cardia plexus	Touch as felt in the internal body	Love, relationships
Third chakra	Solar plexus chakra	Solar plexus	Yellow	Muscular system, integumentary system, digestive system, eyes, face	Pancreas, coeliac plexus	Sight	Perception
Second chakra	Base chakra	Center of abdomen (hara)	Orange	Reproductive system	Gonads, aortic plexus	Taste	Sexuality, basic needs for food and sex
First chakra	Root chakra	Perineum	Red	Lymphatic system, skeletal system, excretory system	Adrenal glands, pelvic plexus	Smell	Trust, survival

 Tips for Passing

Read every possible answer before answering. The last one might be it!

Affirmation

Positive thinking manifests within me in any situation of need.

Practice Questions

1. The chakras are associated with what type of glands?
   a. Sudiferous glands
   b. Sebaceous glands
   c. Epithelial glands
   d. Endocrine glands

2. The chakra that is associated with perception is the _____ chakra.
   a. Heart
   b. Base

    c. Third eye

    d. Solar plexus

3. There are _____ primary chakras.

    a. 5

    b. 7

    c. 6

    d. 8

4. The chakra that is associated with the color green is the _____ chakra.

    a. Heart

    b. Solar plexus

    c. Crown

    d. Base

5. The chakra associated with communication is the

    a. Heart chakra

    b. Third eye chakra

    c. Root chakra

    d. Throat chakra

6. Releasing waste from the body is associated with the _____ chakra.

    a. Crown

    b. Third eye

    c. Root

    d. Throat

7. Chakras are associated with

    a. Emotions

    b. Certain glands

    c. Colors

    d. All of the above

8. The root chakra is associated with the sense of

    a. Smell

    b. Taste

    c. Touch

    d. Hearing

9. Indigo is associated with the _____ chakra.

    a. Throat

    b. Crown

    c. Root

    d. Third Eye

10. The thyroid gland is affected by the _____ chakra.

    a. Throat

    b. Third eye

    c. Crown

    d. Solar plexus

PART 5

Theory, Assessment, and Application

CHAPTER 24

Client History

The study and knowledge of the universe would somehow be lame and defective were no practical results to follow.

—Marcus Tillius

HIGHLIGHTS

Obtaining a thorough client history, also known as an **intake,** is one of the most important parts of being an effective massage therapist. Taking the client's **medical history** serves several purposes. It allows you to find out what the **client expectations** are for the massage, such as relief from a backache or sore neck. It allows you to find out if there are **contraindications** to be observed, such as **disease** or **recent injury.** Finally, the initial client interview gives you time to listen to the client and establish a working rapport.

The intake form should include basic information, such as the client's address, phone number, an emergency contact, and insurance provider, if your office accepts insurance or your client gets reimbursement for your services. An effective intake form can provide you with a lot of insight into the client's general condition and even his or her attitude. The intake form can be customized by the therapist; for example, in addition to questions about the client's medical condition, the form might include such items as "rate the amount of negativity in your life on a scale of 1 to 10" and "rate the amount of responsibility that you take for your own well-being." Many medical print supply companies sell preprinted forms, or you may prefer to make your own.

One of the most important parts of the interviewing process is to obtain **informed consent** from your client for the work you are going to do. Performing a thorough **assessment** will help you decide what type of **care plan** is appropriate. The care plan discussion with your client should include the modalities you are going to use; the recommended frequency of sessions and their length; after-care suggestions, such as stretching exercises or the application of ice—always being careful, of course, not to prescribe or diagnose. The care plan is contingent on the combined goals of client and therapist, whether to relieve pain, restore lost mobility, or assist in injury recovery.

The intake form should include an initial assessment of the client's **posture,** recognizing and recording any **gait** problems or issues with **range of motion,** and any other symptoms, such as numbness or tingling, the client may be experiencing. The postural analysis is an important part of the bodywork session. A full-length mirror is an invaluable tool for showing clients where they are out of balance before receiving the bodywork, and after the session they can see the improvement in the mirror. You may want to use a plumb line, a grid, or something as simple as two pieces of tape crossed on the wall to aid in the postural assessments. To assess gait, ask the client to walk toward you and then away from you. Note whether the client seems to be leaning to one side, walking on the inside or outside of the feet, and so on. If the client reports difficulty with range of motion, you will want to further assess that by performing passive joint mobilizations or asking him to demonstrate for you what range he does have (active joint mobilizations).

During the initial interview, ask what movements are causing problems for the client. Is sitting more comfortable than standing? Does driving cause him pain? On a scale of 1 to 10, how would he describe his level of pain at this moment? Does his work involve repetitive motion? Whether these questions are on the form provided at your office, ask them.

Always allow ample time to talk to your clients, and conduct a thorough interview before working on them. Here is an example of what can happen. A fellow therapist told me she had made an appointment by telephone with an 88-year-old woman. The therapist asked if she was being treated for any medical problems, and the woman said no. When she arrived at the therapist's office, she stated on the intake form that she had high blood pressure in the vicinity of 220/160. The therapist was very concerned and told the client she could not massage her without talking to her physician. The woman's answer was that she was refusing any treatment for the blood pressure, against the advice of her physician, so it would not do any good to talk to him.

What would you do in that situation? What if someone refuses to divulge information? What if they fill out the intake form with nothing but their name and address filled in? Do you assume that nothing is wrong, or do you probe further? What you don't know can hurt you, and the client. If a client outright refuses to fill out the intake form, you'll have to follow your own instinct about whether to perform massage. On the NCE, the correct answer in such a scenario would be no, do not give the client a massage.

If a client lists something on the intake form with which you are not familiar, take the time to call the doctor or at least look it up in a medical reference or in one of the reliable Internet sources, such as a medical school database. An example illustrates this point: A woman reported on the intake form that she has Steven Johnson syndrome. That may sound harmless, but it actually can be life-threatening, and the skin is the primary organ involved. It is a condition of severe blistering, and the skin actually comes off in sheets under even very light pressure. It is usually caused by a reaction to a prescription medication or, sometimes, to an over-the-counter drug. The therapist worked on her, and a couple of days later, the client called to cancel her next appointment. She had a severe inflammation in the neck and shoulder areas and the doctor said it was probably caused by the massage. Sometimes the clients themselves are not a reliable source of information about their own illnesses, as in this case. It is better to call the doctor, or otherwise investigate, when you are presented with something you know nothing about.

You only get one time to make a first impression. Part of the intake process is to set clients at ease and to assure them that you are a professional. In states that have licensure, you are obligated to have your license prominently displayed in your workplace. Be sure your professionalism follows you into the massage room. Use the correct medical terminology if you refer to a body part. You don't have to sound like an anatomy professor, but you do want to give the client the impression that you have been educated and that you are trained and knowledgeable about what you're doing.

SOAP Notes

SOAP notes are used by health care professionals throughout the world to keep track of client/patient progress. Taking a thorough client history is the first step in establishing a file for your client, and SOAP notes should be a vital part of the first and every subsequent visit. There are a number of reasons for keeping careful notes. You cannot expect yourself to remember the details of each client's condition from visit to visit, especially if you are a busy therapist. You may work in a clinic situation in which more than one person sees the same client and have an obligation to share information. More importantly, you cannot expect to get reimbursed by insurance companies, if you are in a position to, unless you are keeping excellent notes. Finally, the law in your state may require it.

A few years ago, licensure for massage therapists was introduced in my state. At that time, therapists who had been practicing for a certain number of years and had proof of performing at least 400 documented massages were "grandfathered" in without having to meet the new requirements for licensure. When I was a massage school administrator, quite a few former students complained about the new law because they had never kept any notes. They certainly had not learned that at massage school! Although I felt badly for them, it was their own fault for not conducting business in a professional manner.

SOAP notes should be a part of your professional duties from your first client visit to the last; they will allow you to chart the client's progress. Having SOAP notes also enables you to provide a more thorough report on their progress. If you have noted things on the first session that have improved by the second or third, you are able to point that out.

SOAP stands for:

- *S: Subjective.* What did the client say? *Example:* Client states sore lower back since returning from hiking trip 3 days ago. Client self-rates pain at 10.
- *O: Objective.* What did you observe? Remember, this is not a diagnosis. This is what you observed through **palpation** (touching, searching with the fingers) and/or postural or other physical analysis. *Example:* Taut bands in medial gluteus, bilateral; trigger points active in gluteus maximus left side. Referred sciatic pain down to knee area.
- *A: Assessment.* What action did you take, and what were the results? *Example:* Myofascial release in lumbar/gluteal area followed by 30 minutes of NMT; reduced pain level from 10 to 4.
- *P: Plan.* What care plan do you suggest for your client? Remember, this is not a prescription. *Example:* Return for another session in 3 days. Suggested epsom salt baths to help soreness.

Use Western medical language and correct anatomical terminology. Your SOAP notes should represent you as a professional therapist. I once read the notes a fellow therapist had previously written on a client I was seeing, and they said: "Fourth chakra spinning wildly backwards." While I am happy to have that information for myself, I don't think the client's insurance company would take the condition seriously. If you are working from a standpoint of **body/mind/spirit,** keep your official SOAP notes confined to the physical, and write notes such as the one presented here on a separate sheet of paper. The same applies to situations in which clients experience a profound or traumatic **emotional release,** sometimes referred to as **somatoemotional release,** on the table. You may want to note that somewhere, but not on the SOAP notes that go to the insurance company. Table 24.1 shows a comparison of proper and improper SOAP notes.

Concerning emotional release, your job as a massage therapist is not to be a psychologist. Your job is to be a compassionate listener and to soothe the client with a nonthreatening, nonsexual touch. Never be in judgment. Don't take on the client's problems or try to solve them. Go ahead and make a referral to a mental health professional, if that's appropriate. Showing concern for the client is your job, but counseling is not.

WHAT YOU NEED TO KNOW

Assessment: a preliminary evaluation before giving a massage; may include a postural assessment, gait assessment, or other physical assessment intended to gain insight into the condition of the client. May also be performed after massage to note improvement.

Care plan: a course of treatment mutually decided on by the client and the therapist with the goals and means clearly stated.

Contraindication: any condition that would be aggravated by receiving massage.

Informed consent: the client's right to know and give permission to receive any treatment; it may be rescinded at any time before or during treatment.

TABLE 24.1 Soap Notes Language	
Proper Soap Notes	**Improper Soap Notes**
S: Client states tension and soreness in shoulders. Works at a desk all day. On a scale of 1–10, pain is an 8.	S: Client feels terrible.
O: Taut bands in rhomboids, bilateral. Left trapezius and levator scapula appear shortened and tender. Left SCM has taut bands.	O: Fourth chakra spinning backwards. A few muscles were tight.
A: NMT effected relief. Pain is now at 2.	A: Did some work on her.
P: Suggested client return weekly for several weeks and demonstrated stretching exercises for her to perform several times per day during work and at home. Suggested she might want to change to a better pillow for cervical support.	P: Come back in 2 weeks.

Intake: the process of taking a thorough health history of the client before proceeding with massage; preferably written, but may be verbal in some circumstances.

Palpation: searching and feeling the body with the fingers.

SOAP notes: a four-part series of notes—subjective, objective, assessment, plan—that records the progress of each session.

 ## Tips for Passing

Prepare for your success and show that self-confidence by sending in your test application immediately, if you have not already done so. If you have done so, then call and schedule the appointment to take the examination. You will then have a concrete goal to look forward to and to help keep you on task. Bear in mind that the turnaround time for your application may be 4 to 6 weeks.

Practice Questions

1. A client comes in and reports that her lower back has been hurting ever since she mowed her lawn yesterday. In which section of the SOAP notes is this information recorded?
   a. S
   b. O
   c. A
   d. P

2. To assist in making a postural assessment, you could use
   a. A plumb line
   b. A grid
   c. Two pieces of tape on the wall
   d. All of the above

3. SOAP is the acronym for
   a. Structure, Objective, Assessment, Protocol
   b. Subjective, Objective, Assessment, Practice
   c. Subjective, Observation, Action, Plan
   d. Subjective, Objective, Assessment, Plan

4. Informed consent should be obtained from each client. You should obtain it
   a. Before doing any work on the client
   b. Before the client leaves the office
   c. After the client has completed one session
   d. While the client is on the table

5. Your client is experiencing pain in the arm, wrist, and hand. You are pretty sure he has carpal tunnel syndrome. You should take the following action.
   a. Share your diagnosis with the client
   b. Apply a heating pad for a short time followed by cryotherapy
   c. Tell him to take a couple of aspirin for the pain, and give him some exercises to do at home
   d. Suggest that he see his doctor for a diagnosis

Affirmation

Today I will rejoice in my abilities.

6. Touching and feeling the muscles for signs of tautness or trauma is referred to as
   a. Effleurage
   b. Palpation
   c. The Knapps technique
   d. Nerve stroking

7. Your client reports that she is suffering from cat scratch fever. She really doesn't have much information on it. You should
   a. Call the doctor before doing the massage
   b. Just go with the limited information she gave you
   c. Call your aunt who has seven cats for advice
   d. Send her home and tell her to come back when she is well

8. Because you were running late, you hurriedly put a first-time client on the table without performing any physical assessments other than quickly looking him over while he filled out the intake form. As you start to work on him you notice his shoes on the floor are very unevenly worn on the outside of the heel. This is a sign that
   a. The feet are inverted
   b. The feet are everted
   c. His latissimus dorsi is shortened
   d. He has calcium deposits on his calcaneus

9. When a client experiences an emotional release on the table, you should
   a. Tell her what happened when you were confronted with the same situation
   b. Act as if nothing unusual is happening
   c. Be present with her and act the part of a concerned listener
   d. Stop the massage; you can't deal with this

10. Subjective information is obtained by
    a. Assessing the way the client walks
    b. Palpation
    c. Standing the client on the plumb line
    d. Listening to the client

CHAPTER 25

Universal Precautions

Education is not the filling of a pail, but the lighting of a fire.

—WILLIAM BUTLER YEATS

HIGHLIGHTS

Universal precautions are procedures practiced by health care professionals that we observe to make massage safe and sanitary. The therapist is obligated to provide a clean and safe environment, including clean linens and drapes for each client. **Draping** is the practice of covering clients properly with sheets or towels to respect their modesty and to provide comfort (Fig. 25.1). Most states with licensure have similar draping laws, requiring that genitals, gluteals, and women's breasts be kept covered. In my state, the drape may be temporarily removed to allow therapy involving the gluteals and breast tissue. Be sure you are familiar with the laws in your particular state.

The client should have the expectation that you wash your hands before and after each massage and during a session, if necessary. If you have to sneeze or cough while performing a massage and you reflexively put your hand to your mouth, excuse yourself to wash your hands. If it is possible to turn away from the table, try to keep both hands on the client's body as you turn your head. If the client is lying in the prone position, she will know that you didn't sneeze into your hand and then put it back on her. Certain diseases are transmitted through droplets that are breathed, sneezed, or coughed through the nose or mouth of an infected person and inhaled by someone else. While you are observing the contraindications of any sores or open wounds on the client, *you* should not be performing massage if *you* have an open wound on your hands or a contagious condition that could affect your clients.

Clients who have chronic conditions may be worked on during nonacute phases

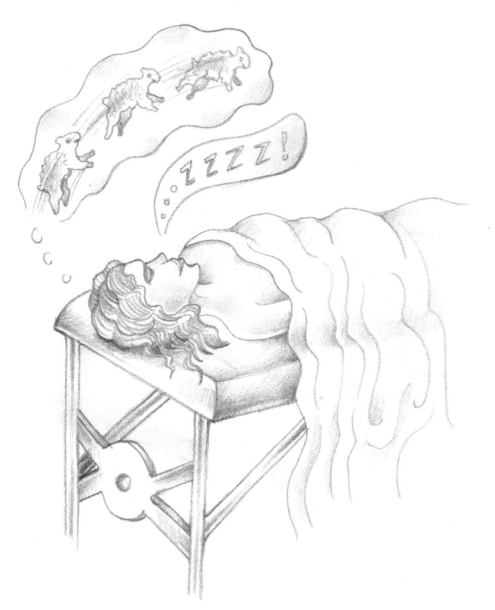

FIGURE 25.1
A properly draped client feels safe and warm and nurtured.

of their illness under a physician's supervision. HIV infection and AIDS are not spread through casual contact. HIV-positive or AIDS-infected individuals can receive massage without any risk of infecting the therapist, as long as there are no open sores or lesions or other contraindications that are a result of their infection, such as pneumonia or extreme distress on vital organs or systems. Again, if a client has any condition that causes you concern, check with his or her physician before doing the bodywork.

Universal precautions should be observed with every client. If you treat all clients as if they are potential carriers of a contagious condition, you won't have anything to worry about. Although in normal circumstances a massage therapist would not be exposed to bodily fluids, you might perform an intra-oral massage to relieve temperomadibular joint (TMJ) dysfunction, which entails placing a gloved hand inside the client's mouth. Many people are allergic to latex, so it's best to use an allergy-free brand of glove for this technique. It is also advisable to wear gloves when performing work on pelvic floor muscles, just as an extra measure of precaution. Washing your hands even after using gloves is necessary, in case the gloves might have been torn or contaminated.

In my state, therapists are obligated to have training in **First Aid** and **CPR (cardiopulmonary resuscitation).** The possession of these skills should be viewed as a universal precaution and obligation for the safety of the client. If your state does not require it, you would be wise to take the course anyway. The basic class prepares you to be a first responder in emergencies—for example, a client experiencing a heart attack on the table, tripping and breaking an ankle on your front steps, or choking on a snack you have in a bowl in the reception area. It goes without saying that for any serious event you are going to call 911, but it's better to be prepared to take some sort of action while you are waiting for the ambulance to arrive. Every minute is precious if someone is in a life-threatening situation.

In a First Aid class I attended, the teacher told a story of someone who had a fainting spell that might have been benign, but the person slumped down against a wall and landed in the floor with his chin on his chest. Not wanting to move him, a bystander called 911. The emergency responders could not revive the person and said he probably would not have died if he had been lying flat on the floor; in the position he was in, his windpipe had been obstructed and he couldn't breathe.

Your office should be a clean, safe haven. Avoid any obstructions on the floor that clients might trip over. If you live in an area prone to snow or ice, keep walkways clear. Smoke detectors and fire extinguishers should be in place. As with any health care professionals, our first obligation is "do no harm." It is our responsibility to ensure the care and safety of all clients. You have in your office the equivalent of a public restroom—different people coming in and out. Keep it spotless, and use a **germicide** for cleaning. Store dirty linens out of view of clients, if at all possible. I use a laundry service and occasionally come across a seemingly clean, folded sheet that appears to have bodily fluid on it. Check your linens carefully; when in doubt, throw it out. If you are washing your own linens, use hot water, an antibacterial detergent and/or rinse agent, such as chlorine bleach, and a hot dryer—these are all necessities. Be sure to wash your hands after handling soiled linens.

WHAT YOU NEED TO KNOW

CPR (cardiopulmonary resuscitation): a procedure for restoring normal breathing to a person with respiratory distress after cardiac arrest; consists of alternating chest compressions and breathing support. Also called mouth-to-mouth resuscitation.

Draping: covering clients with sheets or towels to respect their modesty and provide comfort.

First Aid: actions taken as a first response to injury or sickness, such as applying a tourniquet or administering CPR.

Germicide: a chemical substance containing antibacterial properties used to clean surfaces.

Universal precautions: safety measures practiced by those in the health care professions to prevent the spread of infectious disease.

Tips for Passing

This sounds like common sense, but proofread your examination before hitting the "finish" button. Check for simple errors you may have committed because you were nervous or in a hurry.

Affirmation

I feel a great sense of hope and confidence.

Practice Questions

1. A new client comes in and states in the intake interview that he is HIV-positive. Your response is to
   a. Interview him a little more thoroughly to find out what, if any, complications he has and proceed with the massage in the normal manner, observing all universal precautions
   b. Tell him to go to the doctor and get a permission slip for the massage
   c. Refuse to work on him; you don't want to get HIV
   d. Ask him how he got the condition

2. If you have a bad cold, you should
   a. Go ahead and work, it won't kill you
   b. Call your clients and reschedule them
   c. Blow your nose repeatedly during the massage
   d. Say nothing about it, and maybe your clients won't notice how sick you are

3. A client coughs into her hands several times during the massage session. As a measure of precaution, what should you do before the next client arrives?
   a. Change the linens
   b. Ask the client to get up and wash her hands
   c. Disinfect everything she has touched with a germicide
   d. Offer her a pair of your disposable gloves

4. Universal precautions should be observed
   a. With all clients who have any symptoms
   b. With any client who is HIV-positive
   c. With any client
   d. With any client who has recently been sick

5. A client comes in who has an ugly red rash. She said she hasn't been to the doctor because the rash just broke out yesterday and it doesn't itch, so she doesn't think it's serious. The best course of action is
   a. Put on gloves and give her the massage
   b. Offer her some lavender oil for the rash
   c. Don't worry about it at all, because she isn't concerned about it and it doesn't itch
   d. Politely refuse to massage until she sees the doctor

6. If you sneeze while you are giving someone a massage, you should
   a. Say, "excuse me"
   b. Don't acknowledge it at all; you think they're asleep anyway
   c. Excuse yourself to go wash your hands
   d. Wipe your hand on your shirt

7. You should wash your hands
   a. Before and after you have your lunch break
   b. After handling the laundry at the office
   c. Before and after each client
   d. All of the above

8. It is wise for massage therapists to be trained in CPR and First Aid because
   a. The National Board requires it
   b. They might have to be a first responder
   c. They can't get licensed if they don't
   d. It makes them appear more credible and professional

9. The purpose of proper draping is
   a. To respect the modesty of the client
   b. To protect the integrity of the therapist
   c. To keep the client warm
   d. All of the above

10. If a client tells you that he is not cold or modest and he doesn't need the drape, you should
    a. Take it off of him
    b. Explain that draping is a law, as well as a safety precaution, and you are obligated to abide by that
    c. Act as if you didn't hear him and carry on with the massage
    d. None of the above

CHAPTER 26

Contraindications

Information's pretty thin stuff unless mixed with experience.
—CLARENCE DAY

HIGHLIGHTS

Before performing a massage, there are certain rules you, the therapist, need to follow and actions you need to take. Interviewing the client, observing for contraindications, and adhering to ethical guidelines are the three most important things to consider before performing any bodywork.

A **contraindication** is a condition that could be aggravated by massage. Every therapist should be aware of certain contraindications. If there is any doubt in your mind about performing the massage, contact the client's physician before the appointment. If that is not possible, use your own common sense and observe textbook contraindications, such as those listed in your massage therapy text or a good pathology book (e.g., Ruth Werner's *A Massage Therapist's Guide to Pathology,* second edition, Lippincott Williams &Wilkins, 1998). Common sense will sometimes override the textbook. For example, if a client tells you he is terminally ill and wants a massage, you may want to comply—but the textbook answer is what you need to know for the NCE.

When interviewing clients for contraindications, look for the following:

- Life-threatening conditions
- Contagious conditions
- Acute conditions
- New injuries

In the case of **life-threatening conditions, systemic illness,** or **organ failure,** in which the immune system is seriously compromised, massage could harm the client.

In the case of **contagious conditions,** you do not want to work on someone if you are in danger of catching something and passing it on to the next client, whether it's pneumonia or a common cold. Massaging a person who has a viral infection will intensify his symptoms. In the case of **acute conditions,** if someone is in the worst stage of a condition that may not be a contraindication in and of itself, wait until the acute episode is over before scheduling a massage.

For **new injuries,** here are some guidelines. If the client sprained her ankle a few days ago, she is probably ready for the bodywork. If it just happened a few hours ago, don't do it! Suggest the **RICE** formula: rest, ice, compression, and elevation. If a client is in extreme pain, suggest that she visit her doctor. I once had someone call for an appointment who told me he had been rear-ended in a car accident just 2 hours before and he thought he had whiplash. I suggested he see a doctor immediately.

A good rule of thumb is that if the client is in control of the condition, go ahead and schedule the massage; if the condition is in control of the client, don't. If you are drawn to energy work in its many forms, there are times when massage can't be tolerated but energy work can. That will be for you and your client to decide. If massage is to be part of a post-injury recovery program, communication with the treating physician is vital. People who have sustained fractures should not be worked on until the affected area is completely healed. Muscle and tendon ruptures should not be massaged until at least 48 hours have passed, or longer, depending on the extent of the injury.

Never massage someone who is under the influence of drugs or alcohol. In their impaired capacity, such clients might say or do something inappropriate—or accuse *you* of saying or doing something inappropriate. It goes without saying that *you* should never perform massage while under the influence of drugs or alcohol.

Clients With Special Needs

There are different camps among massage therapists concerning cancer patients. For many years, massage schools taught that cancer was a contraindication, period. The general attitude now is somewhat more relaxed. A person who has a benign tumor on the foot is okay to receive massage on the foot or on other parts of the body. A person with metastatic cancer (cancer that has spread) or cancer involving the immune system is contraindicated. Before performing a massage on any person who is or has been involved in treatment with radiation or chemotherapy, be sure to consult the client's physician.

When radiation has been used to treat bone diseases, it can leave the bone brittle and damaged, and even light touch could cause a bone to break. The same is true of someone with advanced osteoporosis (a loss of bone density). Even light touch could cause a break. Elderly people and people with chronic conditions must be treated with extra caution.

As mentioned in Chapter 24 on client history, there are times when clients are not forthcoming with important information about their health. For instance, maybe a client failed to mention having ringworm and you find it on her body. It could have been in an area she can't see. Or you may be the first to notice a suspicious-looking mole on someone's body. Don't scare the client, but it's your responsibility to mention it. It's up to you to decide whether you will massage any area, the whole body, or none at all if you find something that the client has not divulged.

Pharmacology

Until recently, there has not been much information regarding massage and the possible effects of prescription drugs and their interactions. I recommend a book by Jean Wible titled *Pharmacology for Massage Therapists* (Lippincott Williams & Wilkins, 2004). Wible, who is an RN as well as a massage therapist, has a basic premise: if the drug sedates, the massage should stimulate, and if the drug stimulates, the massage should sedate. Call the doctor when in doubt. Some drugs cause muscular pain as a side effect, and one of the popular cholesterol-lowering drugs is one of them. Clients have told me they felt they had to make a choice between a dangerously high cholesterol level and muscle pain that is so intense they can hardly function—not a good choice to face.

My massage school did not teach pharmacology, and I have noticed through my large collection of massage school catalogs that other schools don't seem to be addressing it either. As massage moves more into the mainstream of the health care professions, pharmacology will be a necessary part of our education. And if it's not addressed in school, conscientious therapists will study it independently.

WHAT YOU NEED TO KNOW

A skilled therapist can often modify bodywork to accommodate most situations, but a physician should always be consulted for the following conditions:

Aneurysm (a sac-like protrusion from a blood vessel or the heart, resulting from a weakening of the vessel wall or heart muscle)

Arteriosclerosis (a chronic disease of the arteries, often caused by plaque or hardening of the arteries because of fibrosis)

Artery blockage, severe

Asthma (a respiratory disease characterized by narrowing of the bronchi, making it difficult to breathe)

Burns (okay after healed)

Cancer that has metastasized or that involves the lymphatic system

Diabetes, if gangrene, insulin shock, coma, or organ failure is present

Failure of vital organs or systems (kidneys, lungs, liver, heart)

Fever (an abnormally high body temperature)

Frostbite (injury from cold causing a loss of circulation and sensation; cells die in the affected area because of freezing of intracellular water)

Hemophilia (a disease characterized by lack of clotting factors in the blood, causing a tendency to bruise easily and bleed freely, even from a minor injury)

High blood pressure, severe

Inflammation

Influenza, acute stage

Open wounds or sores (avoid area)

Periostitis (an inflammation of the connective tissue that covers bone surface except at joints)

Phlebitis (an inflammation of a vein)

Pitting edema (the presence of abnormal amounts of fluid in the intercellular spaces)

Pneumonia (an inflammation of the lungs accompanied by hardening of normally expelled mucus and cellular debris)

Pregnancy with problems (toxemia, ectopic)

Recent surgery (okay after incision heals)

Shock (a sudden metabolic disturbance characterized by failure of the circulatory system to maintain adequate blood flow to vital organs, or a sudden loss of mental equilibrium, usually caused by physical or strong emotional trauma)

Stroke or heart attack if the client is still in imminent danger

Thrombosis (a type of blood clot that causes vascular obstruction)

Less serious conditions may also indicate that it's best to avoid massage. Shingles, hives, poison oak, poison ivy, and other skin outbreaks are contraindications. If a client has a localized injury or infection, such as something on the foot, proceed with the massage with caution, and avoid the traumatized area. Open sores should always be avoided. Any areas of inflammation should be avoided, including bone and joint inflammation. **Periostitis,** for instance, is an inflammation of the sheath covering bones. Light massage can soothe the client, but deep massage will exacerbate the condition. Although heat and redness are general indications of inflammation of soft tissue, an inflammation that is in the bone or the joint is not as likely to be noticed by the therapist. This reinforces the importance of careful intake interviewing and getting clarification on conditions with which you may not be familiar. Varicose veins (a permanent dilation of a vein) should be avoided. There are times when massage could actually cause a fatality—such as dislodging a thrombosis in the calf muscle that could travel up the vein and damage a lung, an event known as pulmonary embolism. Such cases are rare but it could happen, and you don't want it happening to you.

Mental problems are often overlooked as a contraindication. I once had a social worker call to see if I would be interested in working with a schizophrenic patient; he thought massage would calm him down. There's little doubt that it would have, but further investigation revealed the person was delusional. If there is any possibility that the person could be a danger to you or himself, or so delusional that he might perceive that you did something to hurt him or something improper, you will have to refuse. Common sense should dictate, and always err on the side of caution.

Other contraindications to be observed are the body's **endangerment sites,** areas where superficial veins, arteries, nerves, or organs could be damaged by deep massage. Obvious ones are the jugular vein, the carotid artery, the kidneys, and the popliteal triangle (the soft area behind the knee). You won't damage anyone by performing a light stroke over the kidneys, but that's the key—light.

 Tips for Passing

Don't leave the testing center early. You are allowed 3 hours for the examination; take the full amount of time. Careless mistakes and overconfidence can lead to failure. Go back through the test one question at a time, and make sure you have given the best answers.

Practice Questions

1. Your first client of the day tells you she has been taking her own temperature every morning as a means of tracking her ovulation. She tells you she has a low-grade fever this morning, but she isn't worried because she feels fine. You should
   a. Go ahead with the deep tissue massage she is scheduled for
   b. Give her a massage, but make it Swedish so it isn't that deep
   c. Reschedule the appointment
   d. Call her doctor

2. A client with extremely high blood pressure disagrees with her doctor about whether massage is contraindicated and informs you she is going against his advice because she wants the massage. You are going to
   a. Send her home without the massage
   b. Call the doctor before making a decision
   c. Put her on the table and use gentle holding techniques and/or energy work
   d. Have her sign a release for relieving you of any responsibility, and give her a massage

3. The popliteal triangle, an endangerment site, is located
   a. In the hollow of the throat
   b. Superior to the pubic symphysis
   c. Inferior to the mandible
   d. Behind the knee

4. Thrombosis is another term for a
   a. Blood clot
   b. Thyroid disorder
   c. Sore throat
   d. Lung inflammation

5. A client who has had recent radiation therapy may be contraindicated for deep tissue massage because of the effect of radiation on the
   a. Digestive system
   b. Skeletal system
   c. Integumentary system
   d. Muscular system

6. Endangerment sites are places on the body that should be avoided because
   a. The veins are too close to the heart
   b. Organs in the area are subject to inflammation if massage is performed
   c. Veins, arteries, and/or nerves are superficial
   d. A benign tumor is present

7. A regular client confides to you that she recently has had a mental illness diagnosed and has been experiencing intermittent psychotic episodes. Your best course of action is to
   a. Refuse to treat her anymore
   b. Be prepared to subdue her in case she gets violent
   c. Call her doctor (with her permission) to be able to make a more informed decision
   d. Call her doctor (without her permission) to be able to make a more informed decision

8. You should never massage someone who is under the influence of drugs or alcohol because the client
   a. May not be in control of himself
   b. May say or do something inappropriate
   c. May accuse you of saying or doing something inappropriate
   d. All of the above

9. One example of an endangerment site is
   a. Just below the medial malleolus
   b. The axillary area
   c. The maxilla
   d. The occipital ridge

10. A new client refuses to fill out the intake form and tells you that she doesn't believe in doctors or modern medicine. She tells you she hasn't been to the doctor for more than 20 years and claims to have no medical problems. Your best course of action is to
    a. Decline to have her as a client; she may have a condition that is a definite contraindication that has gone undiagnosed because she does not see a doctor
    b. Refer her to another therapist who is not a stickler for following the rules
    c. Conduct a thorough interview, filling out the form as you go along, and check her blood pressure; if it is normal, go ahead with the massage
    d. Proceed with the massage without any further probing

CHAPTER 27

Massage and Bodywork Techniques

If you think of learning as a path, you can picture yourself walking beside her rather than either pushing or dragging or carrying her along.
—POLLY BERRIEN BERENDS

HIGHLIGHTS

Ancient manuscripts and drawings prove that massage was being practiced at least 5000 years ago. The pyramids have hieroglyphs depicting massage and reflexology. Chinese literature documents massage from more than 3000 years ago; the Greeks and Romans practiced massage a few generations later. In the early 19th century, Per Henrik Ling, a Swedish doctor, developed a system of exercise and massage based on physiology and he brought it to the United States. This manipulation of soft tissue came to be known as **Swedish massage.** In 1899, Sir William Bennett opened a department of therapeutic massage at St. George's Hospital in London, validating massage as a useful medical treatment.

The basic techniques of Swedish massage are the foundation for most modalities of Western bodywork. A **technique** is a particular stroke, movement, or pressure applied to the body. *Effleurage,* for instance, is a technique. A **modality** is a system of movements performed in a certain manner with the intent of achieving specific results. Swedish massage, for instance, is a modality. Many times the words *technique* and *modality* are used interchangeably.

Joint Mobilization

Although not massage per se, an important technique for the massage therapist is joint mobilization. **Stretching** and **joint mobilization** are powerful techniques for restoring **range of motion** and **flexibility.** Asking your clients to work through a stretch or mobilization gets them involved in their own care and empowers them to help themselves. Don't wait until the client is on the table to find out about restricted motion; that should be covered on the intake form and during the client interview. The joint mobilizations may be *active*, with the client participating in the motion, or *passive*, with only the therapist performing the motion. The client may provide **resistance** for assisted movements.

Similar procedures are also aimed at increasing mobility and lessening pain. During a **muscle energy technique,** the client actively contracts a specific muscle while in a specific position. During a **positional release technique,** the client is positioned specifically to isolate a muscle, joint, or tendon to effect a release. During a positional release, the client may be asked to perform muscle contractions. Another technique is the **strain–counterstrain technique,** in which the therapist will locate trigger points by palpation, and then assist in positioning the body to lessen pain and reduce muscle strain.

Stretching

Stretches also include techniques similar to those used in joint mobilizations. **PNF (proprioceptive neuromuscular facilitation)** is an active assisted technique in which a muscle is stretched into resistance and then held for 10 seconds, followed by the client holding an **isometric contraction** for 5 seconds, and repeating the process several times. Never bounce during a stretch. Bouncing during stretching is called **ballistic stretching** and should be taboo to a massage therapist; ballistic stretching uses the momentum of a moving limb to try to force it past the point of resistance. Never force a muscle past the point of resistance or past the client's pain tolerance. **Reciprocal inhibition stretching** is an active technique in which the client stretches a muscle and then contracts the antagonist muscle. **Static stretching** may also be active or passive. During either, the muscle is stretched to the point of resistance. In a **passive static stretch,** the client does nothing; the therapist holds the stretch until release is felt. In an **active static stretch,** the client contracts the muscle that is stretched into resistance.

Eastern Techniques

Eastern modalities of massage and bodywork are generally based on meridian theory and often include **acupressure,** a technique of applying pressure with the hands, feet, elbows, and so on, along specific meridian points. Eastern modalities are traditionally performed on a mat on the floor, not on a massage table, although many massage practitioners use modified forms that accommodate the client lying on a table. In Ayurveda and some other Eastern philosophies, massage techniques may be a combination of bodywork and yoga poses and/or stretches, often assisted by the practitioner.

In any form, massage techniques may be performed with the hands but also may use the feet, elbows, forearms, and knees of the practitioner. Some practitioners may also use mechanical devices such as vibrators, percussion instruments (manual or electric), heat lamps, or other machines. Some devices are prohibited in some states, so check the laws in your state before purchasing any mechanical devices. There are also many hand-saving devices, such as T-bars, massage wands, and stones, for use in trigger point work.

Hydrotherapy

Massage and bodywork sometimes includes the use of **hydrotherapy,** the application of water in any of its forms: hot, cold, steam, ice. Each has its own special effects: *thermal, chemical, mechanical,* and *hydrostatic.* **Thermal effects** are produced by the application of water that varies from normal body temperature. The more the treatment temperature varies from normal body temperature, the more effect it will have on the body. The body's internal temperature is normally 98.6°F, whereas skin temperature is normally 92°F. **Chemical effects** occur when water is taken by mouth or used to irrigate a body cavity (which is outside the scope of practice of massage therapy). **Mechanical effects** are produced by the impact of water against the body, such as during a whirlpool bath. When water pressure is exerted on the body surface, it has the **hydrostatic effect** of increasing venous and lymph flow from the periphery and increasing urine output. The application of water also has psychological effects; warmer water is relaxing and soothing, whereas colder water is invigorating and stimulating.

Cold and hot treatments are contraindicated for clients with poor circulation, such as diabetics with peripheral neuropathy. Clients who experience numbness in an area should not receive cold or hot treatments because their lack of sensation would prohibit them from feeling a burn, for instance, if the water or heat pack was too hot. Other contraindications for hot and cold applications include heart disease, lung disease, extremely high or low blood pressure, any major organ infection or failure, and any infectious skin condition. Exceptions should be made only under a doctor's supervision.

Cold Treatments

Applications of cold to the body improve circulation and stimulate the nerves and cells for a short duration. When the application of cold is prolonged, it has a depressing effect on the body. Cellular and nerve functions slow down; blood circulation decreases as the superficial vessels constrict and send blood to the center of the body. When ice is used, it is referred to as **cryotherapy.** The more the temperature of the treatment differs from normal body temperature, the more effect it will have on the body. Cryotherapy is an effective treatment for inflamed areas or areas that are too sensitive for deep work. A short application of ice, or a chemical ice substitute such as a topical spray, may allow the therapist to release trigger points that the client could not otherwise tolerate having touched.

Heat Treatments

Heat has the opposite effects on the body: Blood flow is drawn away from the center of the body to the surface as blood vessels dilate. Once the surface circulation is increased, the blood vessels return the blood to the body's deeper vessels. Heat may be used in the form of moist heat or dry heat. The use of heat also includes saunas, with or without steam. Heat is contraindicated for any areas of inflammation.

Sometimes it is appropriate to use alternating treatments of heat followed by cold. This is particularly true in the case of fibromyalgia, always ending with a cold treatment.

Equipment and Baths

You do not need much in the way of equipment to be able to use hydrotherapy in your workplace. Hot moist towels work just as well as expensive heat packs; they just have to be replaced more often. A convenient method of keeping a supply of ice is to make ice in Styrofoam coffee cups. Then you can just peel away a couple of inches of the Styrofoam, leaving a convenient holder for you to apply the ice to the client. Hot packs or ice packs are sometimes referred to as **fomentations.**

Many spas, health clubs, rehabilitation facilities, and hospitals in which massage is practiced may have expensive equipment on hand, such as **whirlpool baths.** An **immersion bath** may be any temperature. A **sitz bath** normally covers only the hip and pelvic area and is often used to relieve the discomforts of pregnancy, childbirth, hemorrhoids, or other ailments. A **saline bath** includes salt in the water. Many massage therapists routinely advise clients that an epsom salt bath will help relieve muscle soreness.

If you offer retail items for sale in your office, inexpensive hot/cold packs should be at the top of the list. When you recommend to clients that they use a heat pack, for instance, you have it right there on the spot.

Temperatures

- Dangerously hot—110° F or above
- Very hot—105° to 110° F
- Hot—100° to 104° F
- Warm—97° to 100° F
- Neutral—94° to 97° F
- Tepid—80° to 92° F
- Cool—70° to 80° F
- Cold—55° to 70° F
- Very cold—32° to 55° F
- Frozen—below 32° F

Spa Treatments

Spa treatments have become big business, and many massage schools are now addressing spa techniques as part of their regular curriculum. Some techniques involve soft tissue manipulation, whereas others may be nothing more than a topical application followed by a bath or shower. There may be something special about the bath or shower so that it is actually part of the spa treatment as well; a mud bath or milk bath is a good example. Hydrotherapy is often involved in spa treatments in one way or another.

A **Vichy shower** is a multiple-head shower that disperses water ranging from a fine mist to a forcefully directed stream. A **Scotch douche** is extremely forceful hot water that is normally directed along the spine to relax muscles and relieve tension. Although some spa treatments are strictly for the "feel-good" effect, many treatments are therapeutic in nature and often involve massage or reflexology incorporated into the treatment. **Salt scrubs** and **sugar scrubs** are used for **exfoliation** of the skin. Any time the body receives an all-over brushing, regardless of whether products are included, it is referred to as a **shampoo. Herbal baths** or **herbal wraps, mud baths** or **mud wraps,** and many exotic products are now being used in spas for **detoxification** and/or moisturizing.

WHAT YOU NEED TO KNOW

In Swedish massage, strokes are performed toward the heart. It is important to remember that fast strokes (faster than the heart rate) stimulate, whereas slow strokes sedate.

Swedish massage consists of five basic strokes, which are the foundation of most other types of Western bodywork, along with stretching and/or joint mobilizations. The five strokes are:

- **Effleurage:** long gliding strokes in the direction of the heart. The main purposes of effleurage are to get the client used to the therapist's touch, to warm the tissue before doing any deep work, to relax and stretch the muscles, and to increase circulation. Effleurage is also used as a transitional stroke when moving from one body area to another.
- **Pétrissage:** kneading strokes. Pétrissage consists of picking up tissue, kneading, rolling, and lifting. The main purposes of pétrissage are to loosen adhesions, stretch and loosen the muscles and the fascia, strengthen muscle tone, and increase circulation.
- **Friction:** pressure aimed at moving superficial tissue across deep tissue. There are several different types of friction: *circular friction* (small circular movements); *transverse friction,* also called cross-fiber, applied perpendicular to the grain of the muscle; and *pumping,* also called *compression,* applied to the fleshy parts of the body. The main purposes of friction are to loosen adhesions and scar tissue, loosen the fascia, promote flexibility, and improve circulation. Friction may be performed with the thumbs, fingers, palms (called palmar friction), or other body parts, such as the elbows.
- **Tapotement:** percussion strokes. Tapotement consists of slapping, pounding, tapping, hacking, cupping, and pinching. Tapotement stimulates; it is often used at the end of the massage to increase circulation. If applied to the back, it can loosen phlegm in the respiratory tract. Tapotement should be avoided over endangerment sites and injured or sensitive areas, with one exception: tapotement is the recommended stroke for the area of an amputation (providing, of course, that the surgery wound has healed).
- **Vibration:** shaking or trembling movements. Vibration is sedative if applied lightly and slowly, stimulative if applied fast and hard. Rocking and shaking are variations that are also used.

Another stroke, referred to as the **nerve stroke,** is also used at times. It is a very light "feather stroke." It is stimulating and often used to conclude a massage.

 ## Tips for Passing

> It's possible that home may not be the best place for you to study—too many distractions. If that's the case, try the library, the park, or even a coffee shop in the off hours.

Practice Questions

1. To assess a client's range of motion, you could put him through a series of
   a. Nerve strokes
   b. Stretches
   c. Pétrissage
   d. Joint mobilizations

2. To get the client acclimated to your touch and to warm up the muscle, you should begin bodywork sessions with
   a. Effleurage
   b. Friction
   c. Pétrissage
   d. Tapotement

3. A client who has an area of inflammation because of a torn muscle would benefit from
   a. A heating pad
   b. Cryotherapy
   c. Vigorous friction on the inflamed area
   d. Stretching the muscle

4. Ballistic stretching would be the best technique as a treatment for a
   a. Torn rotator cuff
   b. Dislocated patella
   c. Hyperextended neck
   d. None of the above

5. The active assisted technique, in which the muscle is stretched into resistance and then held for 10 seconds, followed by the client holding an isometric contraction for 5 seconds, is the
   a. PNF technique
   b. CNS technique
   c. PNS technique
   d. CNS technique

6. The technique that involves pumping is
   a. Compression
   b. Effleurage
   c. Pétrissage
   d. Vibration

7. The technique that could be used to loosen congestion in the respiratory tract is
   a. Rocking
   b. Pétrissage
   c. Nerve stroking
   d. Tapotement

8. You are gently applying traction to the leg of a client who is lying supine. This is an example of
   a. Active stretching
   b. Passive stretching
   c. Ballistic stretching
   d. None of the above

9. The therapist applying an unassisted stretch to the client would be equivalent to a(an)
   a. Passive static stretch
   b. Ballistic stretch
   c. Passive active stretch
   d. Active static stretch

10. Hydrotherapy has the potential to affect the body in four ways. These are
    a. Chemically, mechanically, thermally, hydrostatically
    b. Active, passive, assisted, hydrostatic
    c. Anatomical, physiological, mental, spiritual
    d. Physiological, pathological, chemical, thermal

CHAPTER 28

Modalities

Education is what you get when you read the fine print. Experience is what you get when you don't.

—PETE SEEGER

HIGHLIGHTS

There are now dozens of modalities of massage and bodywork. A **modality** is a system of movements performed in a certain manner with the intent of achieving specific results. Most Western modalities are based on the five basic strokes of Swedish massage. Many Eastern modalities are based on meridian theory. What separates one modality from another may be as subtle as the amount of pressure applied, or something obvious and out of the norm, like a technique performed only in the water, for instance. Each is unique in some way. Whenever the developer's identity accompanies the name of the modality, it is because he or she is well known in the field, and you should be acquainted with various names. Note that the words *modality* and *technique* are often used interchangeably, as are the words *stroke* and *technique*. The term **stroke** generally refers to one of the five basic techniques (movements) of Swedish massage, which are the basis of most Western modalities (Fig. 28.1).

Some forms of bodywork are intended strictly to release constricted muscles. Others have just as much focus on releasing restricted emotion that may be (in theory) contributing to the pain or discomfort the client is experiencing. These modalities are often referred to as **body/mind/spirit work,** and they are based on the holistic principle that disease ("dis-ease," or out of ease) in one body part causes disease in other parts. There is a lot of overlap among techniques and modalities.

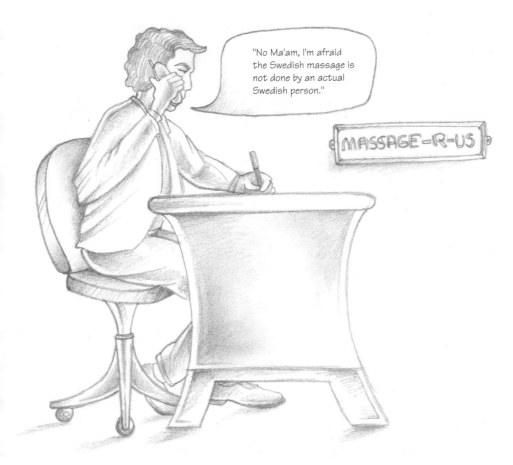

FIGURE 28.1
Identifying modalities by name.

WHAT YOU NEED TO KNOW

Acupressure: using fingers or other body parts to stimulate points along the meridians to facilitate the flow of energy.

Alexander Technique: process of movement re-education to identify and rid the body of faulty postures by replacing habit with conscious movement. Developed by **Frederick Matthias Alexander.**

Amma: traditional Asian massage, sometimes referred to as anma. Using no oil, amma involves stretching, squeezing, and massaging to stimulate the body to become and/or remain healthy; focuses on improving muscle condition and the circulation of ki, or universal life energy. Amma combines bodywork along the meridians with nutrition, detoxification, herbal therapy, and exercise.

Applied kinesiology: the use of muscle testing to evaluate strength and weaknesses or imbalances in the body. Developed by **George Goodhart.**

Aromatherapy: the use of essential oils to restore and to heal.

Aston Patterning: a combination of deep tissue and other massage combined with movement education. Developed by **Judith Aston,** a student of Ida Rolf.

Ayurvedic massage: part of the total Ayurvedic philosophy of health and medicine; techniques that focus on detoxification and the restoration of health.

Bindegewebsmassage: the use of dermatomes (areas of innervation) of connective tissue to identify problems; based on the theory that imbalance anywhere in the body is imbalance in the total body.

Bioenergetics: a combination of breathing, exercise, and psychotherapy aimed at releasing past traumas that are stored in the tissues. Developed by **Alexander Lowen,** a student of **Wilhelm Reich.**

Bowen therapy: a specific series of rolling moves across superficial muscles, tendons, and nerves to stimulate the parasympathetic nervous system into reorganizing areas holding tension or strain.

Breast massage: massage on the breast for the purpose of lymphatic drainage and the prevention (or early detection) of cysts or tumors in the breast and surrounding tissue.

Connective tissue massage: a light technique of dragging and pulling the skin to release the superficial fascia.

Craniosacral massage: a technique that focuses on releasing blockages in the flow of the craniosacral fluid and releasing emotional trauma. **Upledger, Milne,** and **Sutherland** are all known for their respective craniosacral techniques.

Deep tissue massage: Deep pressure massage applied with the fingers, thumbs, elbows, etc., to release the deeper tissues.

Esalen: a body/mind/spirit modality consisting of very light Swedish massage aimed at inducing deep states of relaxation.

Equine massage: an increasingly popular approach of doing massage on horses.

Feldenkrais: a process of unlearning restrictive movement habits and replacing them with efficient, graceful movement. Awareness Through Movement is the movement education part of Feldenkrais. The bodywork part is called Functional Integration, which involves treating the nervous system primarily through the skeletal structure by using hands-on, painless manipulation. Developed by **Moshe Feldenkrais.**

Geriatric massage: a therapy for older adults with attention paid to their specific needs and contraindications.

Hellerwork: a type of bodywork consisting of 11 sessions of structural work combined with vocal work aimed at bringing consciousness to posture and movement. Developed by **Joseph Heller,** student of Ida Rolf.

Hot stone massage: massage performed with heated stones placed and/or rubbed on the body.

Hydrotherapy: the use of water in any of its forms for relaxation or rehabilitation: ice, heat packs, whirlpool baths, wet or dry saunas. The bigger the variance in temperature from that of normal body temperature, the more intense the effects. Some methods also use water pressure, such as Vichy showers and Scotch douche, to relax sore muscles. Many spas are based on hydrotherapy and may include such modalities as salt glow rubs, mud packs, clay baths, seaweed baths, sugaring, and other therapeutic treatments.

Infant massage: massage performed on infants with attention paid to their needs and contraindications.

Kinesiology: the study of muscle movement. Also refers to several different modalities of muscle testing to restore health and balance to the body, sometimes incorporating nutrition and other forms of bodywork.

Lomi-Lomi: massage grounded in Hawaiian spiritual tradition; many different techniques exist, but all are performed in a rhythmic dance usually accompanied by ceremonial music and incorporating ceremonial ritual. **Auntie Margaret** is regarded as the modern authority on Lomi-Lomi, which is said to be 5000 years old.

Lymphatic drainage massage: massage of the lymph nodes and lymph system. Developed by **Dr. Hans Vodder.**

Medical massage: bodywork performed for the purpose of injury repair and rehabilitation from pathological conditions.

Mentastics: the movement part of Trager work, involving the conscious initiation of movement on the part of the client and then allowing the muscle to go to its natural place.

Myofascial release: any method directed at treating restrictions or adhesions in the fascia and muscles.

Myotherapy: trigger point therapy that includes re-education of the muscle. Developed by **Bonnie Prudden.**

Neuromuscular therapy (NMT): a technique directed at returning the body to a state of structural balance; also referred to as trigger point therapy. Developed in Europe by **Leif** and **Chaitow,** popularized in America by **Paul St. John** and **Janet Travell.**

On-site/chair massage: seated massage performed on a fully dressed client, normally in public or corporate settings where full-body massage is inappropriate or impractical.

Orthobionomy: gentle work to release deep tension and restore structural balance; the client is placed in the most comfortable position that alleviates pain, and the therapist works to find the problem from that standpoint.

Orthopedic massage: massage developed from osteopathic techniques, focusing on rehabilitating connective tissue, tendons, ligaments, cartilage, and soft tissue surrounding a bone injury or insult.

Pilates: movement and exercise aimed at lengthening and strengthening muscles. Developed by **Joseph Pilates.**

Polarity: based on the principle that every cell has both negative and positive poles, the use of gentle touch to manipulate the tissue and restore balance; a body/mind/spirit integrative approach.

Postural Integration: a body/mind/spirit modality that incorporates breath work, deep fascial work, and emotional work to restore structural balance to the body.

Pregnancy massage: massage performed during pregnancy, with attention paid to the client's special needs and contraindications of the condition.

Proprioceptive neuromuscular facilitation (PNF): a technique during which a muscle is stretched to resistance and held for 10 seconds, followed by the client contracting the muscle for 5 seconds.

Reflexology: treating the reflex points found on the hands, feet, and ears that correspond to internal tissues and organs.

Reiki: a method in which the practitioner channels universal energy directed at the healing of the client.

Rolfing: deep structural realignment that takes place over the course of 10 sessions. Developed by **Ida Rolf,** it has been used and developed into many other methods by her former students and others.

Rosen method: breathing and relaxation techniques accompanied by rebalancing alignment and increasing flexibility using nonintrusive touching, verbal interaction, and breathing. Developed by **Marion Rosen.**

Rubenfield synergy: a body/mind/spirit approach combining psychotherapy with movements, postures, talk therapy, dreamwork, and other techniques.

Shiatsu: a form of Japanese acupressure traditionally performed fully clothed on a mat on the floor.

Soft tissue release: a sports massage technique aimed at breaking up scar tissue and stretching the muscles. Developed by **Stuart Taws.**

Soma: a body/mind/spirit modality that combines bodywork and psychotherapy; also referred to as psyche-soma.

Sports massage: the massage of athletes, with attention to their special needs and contraindications.

Structural Integration: also referred to as Rolfing; deep structural realignment that takes place over the course of 10 sessions. Developed by **Ida Rolf,** it has been developed into many other methods by her former students and others.

Swedish massage: therapeutic massage focused mainly on relaxation; the five basic strokes are the basis of many other techniques. **Per Henrik Ling** is credited with bringing Swedish massage to the United States.

Thai massage: work performed on the floor that consists of many assisted yoga-like positionings of the body, along with gentle rocking and stretching.

Thalassotherapy: hydrotherapy using heated seawater.

Therapeutic Touch: energy work focused on balancing the body's aura through gentle, above-the-body manipulations of the energy field. Developed by **Dolores Krieger** and **Dora Kunz.**

Touch for Health: a form of applied kinesiology using muscle testing to determine weaknesses in structure. Treatment is to strengthen the weakness and/or release tightness in the opposing side by performing balances on the meridians. Developed by **John Thie, DC.**

Trager: gentle rocking and other nonintrusive movements to facilitate the release of deep physical and emotional restrictions. The hook-up, a natural state of being similar to a meditative state, is used to connect the practitioner with the energy of the client. Developed by **Dr. Milton Trager.**

Trigger point therapy: a technique directed at returning the body to a state of structural balance; also referred to as neuromuscular therapy. Developed in Europe by **Leif** and **Chaitow,** popularized in America by **Paul St. John** and **Janet Travell.**

Visceral manipulation: gentle soft tissue massage of the internal organs to release adhesions.

Watsu: Shiatsu performed in a warm pool of water.

Zero Balancing: treatments performed with the client fully clothed and in a seated position, progressing to a reclining position; focuses on integrating the physical body with the energetic body. Developed by **Fritz Smith.**

Tips for Passing

When studying, don't skip around. Spend each period of study with a goal in mind: "Tonight, I am going to learn the reproductive system."

Practice Questions

1. What do the modalities Trager, Feldenkrais, and Alexander Technique have in common?
   a. They are performed with the client in a seated position
   b. They require a series of 10 sessions
   c. They contain a component of movement on the part of the client
   d. They are variations of Rolfing founded by former students of Ida Rolf

2. What is the best modality for a client who states she is not in pain and just wants relaxation massage?
   a. Structural Integration
   b. Visceral manipulation
   c. Soft tissue release
   d. Swedish massage

3. The modality in which the practitioner channels universal life energy to the client is
   a. Orthobionomy
   b. Polarity
   c. Watsu
   d. Reiki

4. Upledger and Sutherland are both known for their work in which modality?
   a. Reflexology
   b. Touch for Health
   c. Trigger point therapy
   d. Craniosacral therapy

5. The modality that includes therapist-assisted yoga positionings is
   a. Postural Integration
   b. Thai massage
   c. Bindegewebsmassage
   d. Aston Patterning

6. Which modality would be best for a client who desires energy work instead of massage?
   a. Pilates
   b. Structural Integration
   c. Myotherapy
   d. Therapeutic Touch

7. If a client has recovered from a bone injury and needs rehabilitative massage, the best choice for treatment would be
   a. Sports massage
   b. Bowen therapy
   c. Orthopedic massage
   d. Rubenfield synergy

Affirmation

I deserve success beyond my wildest dreams.

8. Auntie Margaret is associated with
   a. Hot stone massage
   b. Craniosacral therapy
   c. Lomi-Lomi
   d. Trigger point therapy

9. A modality aimed at releasing adhesions around the internal organs is
   a. Therapeutic Touch
   b. Manual lymphatic drainage
   c. Visceral manipulation
   d. Trager

10. The person who is credited with bringing Swedish massage to the United States is
    a. Moshe Feldenkrais
    b. Stuart Taws
    c. Per Henrik Ling
    d. Bonnie Prudden

Professional Standards, Ethics, and Business Practices

CHAPTER 29

The Ethics of Massage and Bodywork

One must be a student before one can be a teacher.
—ANCIENT CHINESE PROVERB

HIGHLIGHTS

The **National Certification Board for Therapeutic Massage and Bodywork** has set up its own **Code of Ethics;** many states and massage schools also have their own guidelines that are very similar in nature and wording. **Professional ethics** is defined as *behaving with integrity in a morally acceptable and professional manner.* The purpose of the NCBTMB's Code is to protect and serve the public as well as those in the profession. Conducting one's business in a safe and courteous manner will enhance the profession for all concerned.

The Code of Ethics

Think of The Code of Ethics as a roadmap to a successful client/therapist relationship. The Code states that practitioners who have achieved national certification will do the following:

- Have a sincere commitment to providing the highest quality of care to those who seek their professional services.
- Represent their qualifications honestly, including their educational achievements and professional affiliations, and provide only those services they are qualified to perform.

- Accurately inform clients, other health care practitioners, and the public of the scope and limitations of their discipline.
- Acknowledge the limitations of and contraindications for massage and bodywork and refer clients to appropriate health professionals.
- Provide treatment only when there is reasonable expectation that it will be advantageous to the client.
- Consistently maintain and improve professional knowledge and competence, striving for professional excellence through the regular assessment of personal and professional strengths and weaknesses and through continued education training.
- Conduct their business and professional activities with honesty and integrity, and respect the inherent worth of all individuals.
- Respect the client's right to treatment with informed and voluntary consent. NCTMB practitioners will obtain and record the informed consent of the client, or the client's advocate, before providing treatment. This consent may be verbal or written.
- Respect the client's right to refuse, modify, or terminate treatment regardless of previous consent given.
- Provide draping and treatment in a way that ensures the safety, comfort, and privacy of the client.
- Exercise the right to refuse to treat any person or part of the body for just and reasonable cause.
- Refrain, under all circumstances, from initiating or engaging in any sexual conduct, sexual activities, or sexualizing behavior involving a client, even if the client attempts to sexualize the relationship.
- Avoid any interest, activity, or influence that might be in conflict with the practitioner's obligation to act in the best interests of the client or the profession.
- Respect the client's boundaries with regard to privacy, disclosure, exposure, emotional expression, beliefs, and the client's reasonable expectations for professional behavior.
- Refuse any gifts or benefits that are intended to influence a referral, decision, or treatment purely for personal gain and not for the good of the client.
- Follow all policies, procedures, guidelines, regulations, codes, and requirements promulgated by the National Certification Board for Therapeutic Massage and Bodywork.

Avoiding Ethics Violations

The NCE questions pertaining to professional ethics may be along the lines of different scenarios to test how you would respond. What if you enter the room to give a massage and the client is lying there naked and exposed, having ignored your instructions to be under the sheet? What if a client asks you for a date? If you can use common sense to answer the questions, then you'll do fine.

By the very nature of what we do—placing our hands on unclothed people—we must be very careful to avoid any appearance of **sexual misconduct,** by being professional in dress and behavior, avoiding sexual relationships with clients, and following draping laws.

Conducting your business in an ethical manner is your safeguard against failure. If you are unethical in your business dealings, it will not take long for word to get around, and you will have a problem attracting clients. Pay your bills on time. Give clients fair value for their money. If you advertise $50.00 for an hour, give the client an hour, not 50 minutes. Keep the appointments you make unless it is a dire emergency, such as your own illness. A habit of changing appointments, regardless of the reason, shows a lack of respect and regard for your clients. Their time is just as precious as yours. Maintaining integrity in all your dealings is your path to success.

Standards of Practice

The National Board's **Standards of Practice** are the guiding principles by which massage therapists should conduct themselves and their day-to-day business. The Standards of Practice govern legal and ethical requirements, as well as guidelines about professionalism, confidentiality, business practices, roles and boundaries, and the prevention of sexual misconduct. If you live in a state in which a test other than the NCE is required, your state board probably has a similar code and their own standards of practice. National certification is available to anyone who meets the education requirements and can pass the examination, regardless of whether the NCE is the accepted standard in your state.

Protecting Client Privacy

Treat your clients as if their **confidentiality** is the most important thing. It is. Don't discuss your clients in social situations or with other clients, even if they are related to each other.

Be sure that your client has given **informed consent** for the bodywork. If you work in a clinic situation, explain that there may be the need for **disclosure** with fellow therapists, and obtain consent for that disclosure.

HIPAA (Health Insurance Portability and Accountability Act) laws, enacted in 1996, address several health care issues, including the security and privacy of health data. These federal laws guarantee clients access to their records and govern how medical information may be used, such as prohibiting information obtained from a client for marketing purposes. You are obligated to inform your clients of how their information is protected and maintained in your place of business and to obtain express consent before sharing that information with an insurance company or other third party. Staying informed about current laws and trends in health care is smart business and vital to your own protection in case a client were to file a complaint against you.

Some of the HIPAA laws bring up seemingly minor offenses against privacy, but if you stop and think about it, they do make sense. For instance, HIPAA requires maintaining client records in a locked storage place. That seems reasonable, but there is much more. For instance, HIPAA stipulates that therapists avoid talking on the phone with clients about their problems in the presence of someone else or having client records on your computer screen where others could see them. Discussing treatment with a client in the waiting room where another client can hear the conversation is another infraction of HIPAA laws.

Scope of Practice

Do not prescribe. Do not diagnose. Do not work outside your **scope of practice.** For example, do not perform bone manipulations; those are for chiropractors or doctors. Do not invade the privacy of your clients by asking unnecessary and unrelated questions about their personal life. Do not give unsolicited and/or unqualified advice, and even if advice is solicited, be careful to avoid any appearance of telling people what to do in any way other than something along the lines of "these vitamins have helped me" or "I have been attending AA for 10 years and it has helped me stay sober." Do not try to enroll your clients in marketing schemes or pressure them to buy products. You can sell products in your workplace, but avoid hard-sell tactics, and don't insist that clients buy anything at all.

The Client/Therapist Relationship

The responsibility for maintaining a professional, mutually agreeable **client/therapist relationship** (also referred to as the *therapeutic relationship*) is on you, the therapist. Respect your client's **boundaries.** If a client feels uncomfortable removing certain items of clothing, or does not want to be touched in certain places, even if it's her nose or big toe, you must be respectful of that, regardless of how unusual you think it is. The client always has the **right of refusal.** It doesn't matter if you think her gluteals need to be released; if she objects, you have to honor her wishes. Recognize the fact that there is a **power differential** in the client/therapist relationship. The client is unclothed, vulnerable, lying down. You are clothed, confident, and standing over her. Her comfort and trust in you should be your only concern.

Transference is a phenomenon that may occur when clients become too dependent on the therapist to meet their emotional needs. It refers to the reliving of past interpersonal relationships with which they have unresolved issues. **Countertransference** may occur as the therapist reacts to the client's transference or to the client in general.

Avoid **dual roles.** If you decide you want to date a client, refer that client to another therapist. Friends and family members may take advantage of your good nature by expecting massage free or cheap, or imposing on you to work with them on Sunday afternoon when you were planning to watch the football game. You may have a hard time saying no to those with whom you have relationships, and you may create your own resentment by continually saying yes.

People who are business or professional associates should also be handled with caution as massage clients. Do you feel comfortable massaging your ex-wife's divorce attorney, or the fourth grade teacher who gave your son a low grade on his report card?

If you work solo, it's important to cultivate reciprocal relationships with fellow therapists for referrals you may need to make. Anyone with whom you would have difficulty maintaining a **professional demeanor** should be referred to another therapist.

Do not practice discrimination. Healing through touch should be blind to race, color, religious affiliation, gender, sexual preference, and ethnicity.

Communication

Communication skills are a necessity for anyone who wants to work with the public. Take your cue from your client. If she wants to talk, fine, but is she is doing nothing more than answering your direct questions, be quiet and let her relax. Clients may say more than you want to hear. Don't get invested in their problems, and certainly do not tell them yours.

Conflict Management

Another obligation of the therapist is developing skills in **conflict management.** If a situation arises between client and therapist or therapist and peer that causes concern, the ideal is to reach a peaceful resolution that will harm none of the parties involved. Perhaps you find a client has unreasonable expectations for the bodywork, or a co-worker is doing something that doesn't suit you, such as expecting you to do all the laundry just because she has more clients than you do. Many books on ethics contain "fire drills"—ethical scenarios that might occur—to help learning in this area. It's hard to know what you'll do in a situation until you're actually confronted with it.

Mentors and Peer Support

Finally, it is a good idea to have a **mentor,** an older, more experienced therapist you can call on for advice and supervision when situations arise in areas in which you are less experienced. **Peer support** is another good idea. Network with your fellow therapists by joining the local chapter of the AMTA or by just getting together with others informally. My peer group shares information and moral support over lunch one Saturday per month. Our monthly gatherings get us out of our own offices and give us all a little time to unwind. Rather than viewing other therapists as the competition, make a choice to view them as colleagues for sharing, learning, and networking.

WHAT YOU NEED TO KNOW

Code of Ethics: guidelines for morally acceptable and professional behavior.

Communication skill: the ability to communicate effectively; a therapist's ability to communicate mutually with clients regarding goals, treatments, outcomes, after-care, etc., and to educate the public about massage.

Confidentiality: respect for the client's right to privacy.

Countertransference: the feelings of a therapist toward a client; the response of the therapist's unconscious toward the transference of the client.

Disclosure: the sharing of personal information (should only be done with permission).

Discrimination: treating a person unfairly due to sex, race, gender, religion, ethnicity, or other reasons.

Dual roles: assuming two roles in relation to the same person; in addition to being a client's therapist, also being a friend, lover, social acquaintance, employee, etc.

HIPAA laws: the laws of the Health Insurance Portability Accountability Act, including specific guidelines that relate to the client's right to privacy.

Morals: the belief system that defines behavior within legal and ethical parameters. A behavior may be immoral and still be legal.

Right of refusal: a client's right to refuse any part of treatment, even if previous permission has been given.

Transference: a client's feelings toward a therapist, often based on fantasy and/or memory or feelings and attitudes toward another person in the past.

Sexual misconduct: any action or verbalization of an inappropriate sexual nature toward a client.

Standards of Practice: the guiding principles by which massage therapists should conduct themselves and their day-to-day business.

Tips for Passing

Think of the examination as an opportunity to succeed at something that is important to you.

Affirmation

It is safe for me to realize my dreams.

Practice Questions

1. A married couple who has been your weekly clients is divorcing. They continue to see you (separately, of course), and each one is pumping you for information about the other: what they said, who they are seeing, and other questions. Your appropriate response is to
   a. Dismiss them both as clients
   b. Dismiss one of them and keep the other
   c. Enjoy the gossiping back and forth
   d. Tell them both politely that your Code of Ethics prohibits you from such behavior, and in the interest of keeping your client/therapist relationship, you are not going to talk about the other

2. A new client is flirtatious during the initial intake interview and asks if you are married. Your best course of action is to
   a. Tell him in no uncertain terms that you do therapeutic massage and do not have personal relationships with clients or share personal information
   b. Tell him the conversation is making you uncomfortable and you think he would be better off going elsewhere
   c. Tell him you feel sick and won't be able to give him a massage after all
   d. Flirt back and pursue the relationship

3. You have instructed your new client to undress and be under the drape in the supine position when you return. Instead, you enter the room to find her naked and sprawled on top of the covers. Your reaction is to
   a. Step back behind the door where you can't see her and loudly say that you'll be in when she gets under the sheet
   b. Just go on in and get to work
   c. Take another sheet in with you and cover her up
   d. Start quarreling with her about her failure to follow directions

4. A client constantly complains of stress. However, you have noticed when he is talking to you that all of his stress seems to be self-induced by taking on other people's problems. Your course of action is going to be
   a. Nothing; just listen and nod
   b. Gently point out to him that he is trying to play the martyr
   c. Suggest he seek counseling for the stress
   d. Suggest he ask his doctor for some Valium

5. A new client starts telling you about her last experience with massage, which was not a good one. She states that the therapist made a sexual overture to her and calls him by name. You happen to know this therapist very well and cannot imagine that he would do such a thing. You should
   a. Tell her she must have been mistaken
   b. Call him immediately after the session to discuss the matter, without divulging the client's name

   c. Call him immediately after the session to discuss the matter, tell him who said it, and exactly what she said

   d. Tell her to report him to the state massage board

6. When a client discusses personal matters with you, what should you do?

   a. Just listen and be compassionate

   b. Offer the client your advice

   c. Tell the client you'd prefer he didn't talk

   d. Tune out the client

7. A new client has left her bra on. Without saying anything to her about it, you unsnap it while she is in the prone position so you can work on her back. You have just violated

   a. The scope of practice

   b. Her morals

   c. Her boundaries

   d. The rules about sexual misconduct

8. A client of yours starts asking you personal questions about another client that she saw leaving as she was coming in. You should

   a. Answer her questions honestly

   b. Tell her politely that you cannot talk about your clients, and that you wouldn't talk about her

   c. Just change the subject

   d. Tell her she is being rude and nosy

9. Another massage therapist has moved into your neighborhood, and you have discovered that she is not licensed. The best course of action is

   a. Send a formal complaint to the licensure board

   b. Ignore the situation; your clients are loyal and you don't have to worry about it

   c. Change your sign to state "The only licensed therapist in the area"

   d. Call her and inform her that you are going to put her out of business

10. A well-known professional athlete lives in your hometown and frequents your business. You just can't help bragging about it. You have violated

   a. The rule of confidentiality

   b. The rule of communication

   c. The Scope of Practice rules

   d. The Standards of Practice

CHAPTER 30

The Business of Massage

The first and most important step toward success is the feeling that we can succeed.

—Nelson Boswell

HIGHLIGHTS

What are you planning to do when that license is finally in your hands—work for someone else or go into business on your own? There are advantages and disadvantages to both. Many massage therapists choose to be self-employed. You may decide to work out of your home, providing it is legal to do so in your locale. You might decide on a have-table-will-travel business, doing on-site massage in the homes and offices of other people. You can rent space, start your own practice, and go to work. Some massage therapists work in hospitals, chiropractic offices, and physician's offices in conjunction with physical therapists, psychologists, or other health care providers. Others prefer more relaxation-focused settings such as spas, salons, resorts, or cruise ships.

Employee or Independent Contractor

If you choose to work for someone as an **employee,** you will probably be on a regular pay schedule and could also receive a percentage of the fees from the work you do. Laundry service is provided by the employer, taxes will be deducted from your paycheck, and other benefits, such as insurance, vacation pay, or company meals, may be provided.

If, instead, you make an arrangement with someone to work in his or her office, for mutually agreed-on terms and hours, and give that person a percentage of your earnings, you are an **independent contractor.** As an independent contractor, you are self-employed. You may be obligated to provide your own massage table, sheets, cream or oil, and other supplies. Clients may be referred to you or scheduled for you during your agreed-on work hours.

Whether making a commitment to be an employee or an arrangement to be an independent contractor, it is essential to get the terms spelled out in writing—your responsibilities, their responsibilities, the expectations for both parties under the agreement. No detail is too small. Here are some of the potential questions that need to be answered to the satisfaction of both parties:

- What is the pay for the job? Is it hourly, or a percentage, or are you paying rent for the space?
- What are the expected days and hours of the job?
- Is overtime required?
- Is there a dress code?
- Are personal items, such as mementos and artwork, allowed in the workspace?
- Are there set break times?
- How much time between appointments?
- Is massage cream or oil provided, or does the therapist provide it?
- Is advertising provided?
- Who is responsible for cleaning the office and/or treatment rooms?
- Are business cards and brochures provided, or are they the individual therapist's responsibility?
- Does each therapist have to pay liability insurance or is there a blanket policy for the business?
- Is there office support?
- Who makes the appointments, you or a receptionist?

Paying Taxes

As an independent contractor, you will be responsible for paying quarterly estimated taxes, including state and federal income taxes, Social Security tax, and self-employment tax (Table 30.1). If you open your own business, you may also be required to file other forms and pay other taxes, such as sales tax if you sell products. If you employ others to work for you, you will have to collect and pay federal, state, and Social Security taxes and may be obligated for other things as well, such as state unemployment tax.

The Business Plan

If you are going to open your own business, it is imperative that you sit down and write out a **business plan.** Even if you aren't ready to go to the bank to borrow the money to finance the business, you still need a plan. The business plan contains expenses for starting and maintaining your business, as well as your **goals** for the coming year. You may want to expand it into a 5-year plan or even a 10-year plan. What do you hope to accomplish, and how are you going to do it? Are you going to spend money to advertise or depend on word of mouth? Use a linen service or wash sheets every night? Give your clients water out of the tap or use a water service? There are many details to consider. A visit to your local Small Business Administration will usually provide you with information about what you need to know about starting your own business, including a list of required licenses and taxes.

TABLE 30.1 Tax Forms

Forms	Who	Why
W-2	Employee of a company	Year-end wage and tax statement to submit with individual's tax return
1099	Independent contractor	Year-end wage and tax statement to submit with individual's tax return for any independent contractor wages in excess of $600.00; equivalent to the W2 form
Schedule K-1	Member of a business partnership in a company	Year-end wage and tax statement to submit with individual's tax return; equivalent to the W2 form
1040	Individual	Year-end tax return form; must be mailed by April 15
1040ES	Self-employed individual	Used for estimated quarterly tax, must be submitted on April 15, June 15, September 15, and January 15th
Schedule C	Sole proprietor of a business	Business profit and loss form for year-end tax return
Schedule SE	Self-employed individual	Self-employment tax form attached to the 1040 form

The business plan will include a **budget.** Table 30.2 shows a sample of a monthly budget. On your budget, you should list all expenses you expect, as well as a miscellaneous category to cover things that you don't expect, like a broken water pipe in the bathroom, plus all revenue you expect to take in. For the first year, that will be a projection with no past history to base it on, so be realistic. You may want 25 clients per week, but what if you only get 10? Can you still make your budget work? What if you are sick and miss 2 weeks of work? Can you still pay your rent? Too many businesses (of every kind) fail because the owner starts out with a big dream and no business plan. After figuring the cost of running your business for 1 month, divide that figure by the price you charge for a massage to reach your break-even point.

Example: If your monthly expenses total $1000.00, and you are charging $50.00 for a massage, you must do 20 massages to break even and pay your bills. Whatever income you receive above and beyond the revenue from 20 massages is your paycheck.

In addition to the expenses listed in the Table, there are payments that are not due every month, such as quarterly payments for renter's insurance; annual payments for AMTA dues and insurance; payments for continuing education, license renewals, and other things that arise, such as the need for new business cards or brochures. Adding another $50.00 per month to cover those items, the monthly total comes to $1500.00. If you have 50 appointments in a month at $50.00 each, you have **gross income** of $2500.00, leaving a **net income** of $1000.00 for the month. Don't forget to set aside the appropriate portion of every dollar for taxes.

Keeping Accurate Business Records

It is essential to keep accurate **business records.** If you have a computer and good business software, you'll be fine, as long as you use them properly. If you are not

TABLE 30.2 Sample Monthly Budget for a Massage Therapy Business		
Monthly Expenses		**Monthly Gross Income 2500.00** **− Expenses 1450.00**
Rent	$725.00	
Electricity	75.00	
City Water	25.00	
Linen Service	140.00	
Telephone	250.00	
Bottled Water	25.00	
Advertising	100.00	
Office Supplies	50.00	
Janitorial Supplies	10.00	
Bank Service Charges	10.00	
Credit Card		
Machine Lease	40.00	
	1450.00	
Net Income		1050.00

computer-savvy, a good pencil and a financial journal, obtainable at any business supply store, will do just as well. Every expense is a potential **tax deduction** for your business, and you will need deductions to offset your income. The **paper trail** is your proof of legitimate business expenses, so save every receipt. If you attend a CEU workshop, staple your payment receipt to the brochure from the class. **Documentation** is key if your tax returns are ever audited.

Recognize your own abilities. You may be a wonderful massage therapist but a poor record-keeper. If you are a person who can't balance a checkbook or do math, hire someone to help you. It might be an easy trade; you may be able to barter with an accountant for bookkeeping in exchange for massage. There are a lot of business services that specialize in small businesses, and they may do a month of bookkeeping for you for less than the price of one massage. Even if you are capable of keeping your own business records, an initial consultation with a tax professional when you are starting out is a good idea; you can find out exactly what forms you are responsible for filing and when. Everyone's circumstances are different, and consulting a professional who deals with these matters daily makes good sense.

Insurance

Accurate records are also essential for client-related paperwork, particularly if you plan to provide services that are eligible for **reimbursement** by insurance companies. Knowledge of **diagnosis codes** (provided by the doctor; remember, massage therapists don't diagnose) and **procedure codes** is a must. SOAP notes, intake forms, and progress notes will all be required by the insurance company, along with other items such as a disclosure form, any payment information, accident reports, a **worker's compensation** form if it's that type of case, a practitioner's lien— there is a lot to consider. A **practitioner's lien** is a legal document that should be signed by the client, the therapist, and the attorney, if one is involved; it is an acknowledgment that the client is responsible for the money owed to you for treatment, in the event that the insurance company does not pay.

Accepting insurance in your massage practice is a guarantee of a certain amount of business; however, can you afford to wait to get reimbursed to get paid? You will want to examine your own financial situation and decide what percentage of money you could wait a while to receive. Some insurance companies are slow to pay, even if you have previous approval to perform the procedure. Illegible records will be turned down for payment. SOAP notes should be written in anatomical terminology (e.g., taut bands in scalenes and SCM; not tight neck). There are services that will file insurance claims for you for a fee; it may be worth it to pay for their experience in handling claims, especially if you are just starting your business.

Liability insurance may not be required for you, but you are wise to have it. If you are working as an employee, getting your own insurance may not be an issue if your company has a blanket policy covering all employees. If you are working on your own or as an independent contractor, you will need to pay for your own insurance coverage. Inexpensive insurance is available through the AMTA, ABMP, and the AMC. Many other specialty associations, such as the International Reiki Practitioners Association, and the International Reflexology Association also offer inexpensive coverage. If your table collapses under a client or a client trips over a loose tile in the bathroom, you will be covered. The peace of mind is worth far more than the price of the policy.

Relationships With Other Professionals

You may be fortunate enough to have other health care providers referring clients to you. If that is the case, they certainly deserve a letter of thanks, as well as follow-up progress notes. Failing to communicate could cost you further referrals. Make an effort to establish professional relationships with every other professional you can: doctors (MD), naturopaths (ND), chiropractors (DC), physical therapists (PT), and mental health professionals (e.g., MD, PsyD). Not only will they be sources of referrals to you but also will there be times that you are in the position of needing to refer a client elsewhere as well. You will also want to cultivate relationships with other massage therapists, especially those who have specialties other than your own. Viewing other massage therapists as colleagues, rather than competition, is a good attitude to have.

The Legalities of Massage

In addition to your national and/or state certification, you may be required to have a state and in some instances a county or township license. You may also need a specific license from your state Department of Revenue. In my state, massage therapists are obligated to maintain a state license as well as a separate privilege license, and some localities require their own separate license. All your credentials should be posted in plain sight where your clients (and the state massage board, should a representative decide to pay you a visit) can see them.

CREATING A HEALING SPACE

Setting the stage for massage in a way that combines professionalism with comfort will enhance your business. Your reception area should be welcoming to the public, with a couple of chairs or a sofa, and magazines for people who are waiting. Every inch of your space—including the reception area, the treatment room, the bathroom, and any other rooms on the premises—should be clean and uncluttered. Be sure your restroom is always stocked with soap, toilet paper, and paper towels and that it is cleaned daily. A cluttered or dusty room is not a place where clients want to spend time.

Music in the massage room should be nonintrusive and played at a soothing volume. Lighting should be soft and not glaring in the client's eyes. Freshly laundered linens, a warm blanket, and a comfortable room temperature are all necessities. Plan to provide a simple one-size-fits-all robe in your office in case a client needs to get up and use the bathroom in the middle of a massage.

Those therapists who work in their homes should be especially conscious of the environment. Although there is nothing wrong with having personal mementoes in your workspace, your child's toy truck should not be blocking the way to the table. You may want to reconsider working in your home if you have a child who is still at the screaming stage.

Your personal hygiene is of paramount importance. Be clean, and use only deodorants that do not have scent added to them. Avoid perfumes and colognes. Be conscious of the personal products you use, especially items that come from a spray can. Hairspray and some cosmetics may have strong odors. Pure organic essential oils are usually acceptable, because they don't contain the synthetic chemicals that irritate people with sensitive sinuses, but even these should be used with caution. Don't use overwhelming incenses or diffuse very strong-smelling oils in your treatment room. Keep your nails trimmed short and remove any hangnails or rough spots on your hands. Obviously, you can't expect clients to relax if you are touching them with something that feels like sandpaper.

Dress in neutral manner. If you like to work in jeans, that's fine, as long as they're clean.

WHAT YOU NEED TO KNOW

Balance sheet: a basic financial statement, usually accompanied by disclosures describing the basis of accounting used in its preparation; lists a company's assets, liabilities, and the equity of its owners. Also known as a statement of financial condition.

Corporation: a form of doing business, characterized by the limitation of the owner's liability to the amount invested in the business.

DBA: "Doing Business As." A form of doing business, usually used by sole proprietors; protection of personal assets is less than when conducting business as a corporation. Example: Tom Smith D/B/A Therapeutic Massage Associates.

Disbursement: a payment by cash, check, or credit card.

Independent contractor: an individual who contracts to work for another, with certain stipulations and no benefits that would be afforded to regular employees.

Mission statement: a written statement of a business's purpose and goals.

Partnership: a business arrangement between two or more people.

Reciprocity: the practice of one state recognizing credentials from another by mutual agreement.

Sole proprietorship: a business arrangement that has only one owner, the sole proprietor.

Target market: the segment of the population for which the advertising and outreach strategies of a business are intended.

Third-party reimbursement: a payment received from an entity other than the consumer, such as an insurance company, the government, or an employer.

 Tips for Passing

If at all possible, give yourself a break and take a day or two off from studying right before the test. An enjoyable day trip or a weekend away should be your reward for studying hard and preparing to pass. Give yourself the gift of a nice break, and you'll feel restored and refreshed when you go to take the test.

Practice Questions

1. If you are working as an independent contractor, the IRS requires that you file quarterly
   a. Sales tax
   b. Self-employment taxes
   c. 1099
   d. 1040

2. If you are a business owner who employs other therapists, pays them by the hour, and provides them with benefits, you will be giving them a _____ form at the end of the tax year.
   a. W-4
   b. WC
   c. W-2
   d. W-3

3. An independent contractor who works in your office comes to work looking sloppy and upset and says that her boyfriend broke up with her last night. She is teary-eyed and not likely to do a good job today. The best course of action is to
   a. Get another therapist to cover her appointments if at all possible and send her home
   b. Fire her on the spot
   c. Cancel her appointments without divulging the reason
   d. Do nothing and let her carry on

4. A written expression of the goals and purpose of a business is referred to as
   a. An advertisement
   b. A business plan
   c. A mission statement
   d. A general journal

5. To protect yourself from a lawsuit, you should have the following
   a. National certification
   b. A state license

   c. A prescription from the doctor to do massage on anyone

   d. Liability insurance

6. What is the main purpose of a code of ethics?

   a. To satisfy the licensure laws

   b. To provide parameters for a safe and comfortable client/therapist relationship

   c. To impress clients

   d. To keep the massage board happy

7. If a massage practitioner who has a license in one state moves to another state and a license is granted based on the license from the previous state, what is that called?

   a. Reciprocity

   b. Equality

   c. Right to license

   d. Dual licensure

8. If a practitioner receives a referral from a doctor, what follow-up form should she provide to the doctor?

   a. The intake form

   b. 1099

   c. Progress notes

   d. The insurance form

9. If you are the sole owner of a business, that is referred to as a

   a. Proprietorship

   b. Partnership

   c. C corp

   d. S corp

10. Which of the following would be legitimate tax-deductible business expenses?

   a. The cost of continuing education after you have your license

   b. Training for a new career in massage therapy

   c. An hourly rate for your time while studying for the licensure examination

   d. Car expenses for commuting to massage school

Answer Key

Chapter 3 Practice Questions

1. **b** The basic unit of human life is the cell.
2. **d** The study of the structure of the body is called anatomy.
3. **c** Cephalad means toward the head.
4. **d** Antibodies are molecules of proteins that are the primary defense of the immune system.
5. **a** Etiology is the study of the cause and origin of disease.
6. **d** The condition characterized by swelling, heat, redness, and pain is known as inflammation.
7. **a** In the Western anatomical position, the human body is standing erect, facing forward, arms at side, palms facing forward.
8. **d** The pericardial cavity is located within the thoracic cavity.
9. **a** The study of the tissues of the body is called histology.
10. **b** A short, severe episode is called acute.

Chapter 4 Practice Questions

1. **b** Contra = against
2. **c** Eryth = red
3. **d** –oma = tumor
4. **c** Arthro = joint
5. **c** Angio = vessel
6. **b** Ab = away from
7. **b** Macro = big

8. **a** –ism = condition of
9. **b** Myo = muscle
10. **c** Nephro = kidney

Chapter 5 Practice Questions

1. **b** The body contains 26 chemical elements.
2. **b** Aluminum is an example of a trace mineral.
3. **b** Electrolytes are substances that break apart into two or more ions when put into water.
4. **a** When in balance, the body's pH should be between 7.35 and 7.45.
5. **c** Free radicals cause tissue damage.
6. **c** An ion is an atom that could be either positively or negatively charged.
7. **d** Chemical imbalances contribute to many conditions, including depression, diabetes, and cancer.
8. **d** Protons, neutrons, and electrons are all examples of subatomic particles.
9. **d** Excess calories are stored as fat.
10. **d** Oxygen, carbon, hydrogen, and nitrogen account for about 96% of the body's mass.

Chapter 6 Practice Questions

1. **d** The study of the structure of cells is called cytology.
2. **a** Energy for many of the body's processes is supplied by ATP.
3. **a** The genetic information of cells is encoded in DNA.
4. **d** Most chemical activities of the cells take place in the cytoplasm.
5. **c** The splitting of a compound into fragments by adding water is called hydrolysis.
6. **d** Organelles are special structures in the cell that perform specific functions.
7. **a** Mitosis results in two daughter cells.
8. **a** Lou Gehrig's disease is also known as amyotrophic lateral sclerosis.
9. **c** People of African descent are affected by sickle cell anemia.
10. **c** Genetic information is transferred from DNA to the cytoplasm by RNA.

Chapter 7 Practice Questions

1. **d** Too much carotene in the body causes the skin to appear orange-tinted.
2. **b** The study of the skin and its pathology is called dermatology.
3. **b** The sebaceous glands form oil.
4. **c** The skin aids in the synthesis of vitamin D.
5. **c** Perspiration is formed by sudiferous glands.
6. **b** The most superficial layer of the skin is the epidermis.
7. **a** Melanin is a pigment produced in the skin that contributes to skin color.
8. **c** A lack of oxygen in the blood causes cyanosis.

9. **d** *Candida albicans* is a fungus.

10. **d** Scleroderma is skin that has hardened.

Chapter 8 Practice Questions

1. **d** The human body has 206 bones.

2. **a** An example of a long bone is the femur.

3. **b** The hyoid is an irregularly shaped bone.

4. **b** The joint where two bones meet is called an articulation.

5. **a** Immovable bones are classified as synarthrotic.

6. **c** An example of a freely moveable joint is the hip.

7. **a** The joint functions as a fulcrum.

8. **c** The most plentiful levers in the body are third class.

9. **c** A meatus is a canal.

10. **d** The coronal and sagittal sutures meet at the fontanel.

Chapter 9 Practice Questions

1. **c** The point where muscle attaches to the moving bone is referred to as the insertion.

2. **c** The connective tissue that binds muscles together is the fascia.

3. **a** Lack of oxygen to the muscle causes ischemia.

4. **b** RICE is the acronym for rest, ice, compression, elevation.

5. **c** The fleshy part of a muscle is the belly.

6. **b** Muscular dystrophy causes a progressive loss of muscle fibers without any nervous system involvement.

7. **a** Muscular atrophy is a progressive weakening of the muscle caused by degenerating neurons.

8. **c** The study of the muscular system is called myology.

9. **d** The condition in which the tendon sheath is inflamed is called tenosynovitis.

10. **d** There are 630 muscles in the human body.

Chapter 10 Practice Questions

1. **c** The nervous system includes two separate systems, the CNS and the PNS.

2. **c** The autonomic nervous system is part of the peripheral nervous system.

3. **b** Neurology is the study of the nervous system.

4. **a** Neurotransmitters are chemical messengers.

5. **c** The two ends of the neurons are called the axon and the dendrites.

6. **d** The space between two cells is called the synapse.

7. **c** Dopamine is both a hormone and a chemical transmitter.

8. **a** The myelin sheath is a layer of insulation surrounding the neuron.

9. **d** There are two main types of cells in the nervous tissue, neurons and glial tissue.

10. **c** Endorphin is a natural opiate produced by the brain to diminish pain.

Chapter 11 Practice Questions

1. **d** It is estimated that the human brain contains around 100 billion neurons.
2. **c** Intelligence, reasoning, and emotion are facilitated in the association area of the brain.
3. **b** Wernicke's area of the brain interprets speech.
4. **a** There are 31 pairs of nerves arising from the spinal cord.
5. **a** The meninges include spinal and cranial meninges.
6. **d** Past sensory experiences are stored in the somatosensory association area.
7. **c** The part of the brain associated with long-term memory is the hippocampus.
8. **d** Melatonin and serotonin are produced in the pineal gland.
9. **c** The protective layer that keeps most substances from penetrating through to the brain from the blood is the BBB (blood–brain barrier).
10. **c** The long tubules extending from the pia-arachnoid that act as one-way valves for the cerebrospinal fluid are the arachnoid villi.

Chapter 12 Practice Questions

1. **c** Cerebrospinal fluid contains glucose and protein.
2. **a** The craniosacral system includes nerves that control the parasympathetic division of the ANS.
3. **c** The membrane that covers the brain and the spinal cord has three layers.
4. **c** Dura mater means tough mother.
5. **d** The craniosacral nerves are involved in the secretion of bile, relaxing sphincter muscles, and the erection of sex organs (among other things).
6. **b** The arachnoid is made of collagen and elastic fibers.
7. **c** Craniosacral rhythm refers to the rise and fall of the cerebrospinal fluid.
8. **c** The pia mater is the inner dural membrane.
9. **b** The subdural space contains interstitial fluid.
10. **b** The epidural space is between the dura mater and the wall of the vertebral canal.

Chapter 13 Practice Questions

1. **a** Hormones are composed primarily of proteins and steroids.
2. **d** The fight-or-flight reflex is controlled by the adrenal glands.
3. **b** Estrogen regulates the sex drive in females.
4. **c** Sex cells are also called gametes.
5. **c** Insulin is secreted by the pancreas.
6. **c** HGH is the acronym for human growth hormone.
7. **c** The general adaptation syndrome is also known as the stress response.
8. **a** The female gonads are the ovaries.
9. **c** The body's metabolism is controlled by the thyroid.
10. **b** If a person is thirsty all the time and has to get up many times during the night to urinate, he or she may have diabetes insipidus (but of course, we are not going to diagnose anything.)

Chapter 14 Practice Questions

1. **b** The body's main line of defense against infection or illness is the leukocytes.
2. **a** There are eight different blood types.
3. **c** The largest artery in the body is the aorta.
4. **c** The smallest blood vessels that carry oxygenated blood are the capillaries.
5. **a** A complete shutdown of the heart is a cardiac arrest.
6. **d** A genetic condition that results in a lack of clotting factors in the blood is hemophilia.
7. **d** Hypertension is the condition of high blood pressure.
8. **d** An excessively rapid heartbeat is called tachycardia.
9. **c** Atherosclerosis is a progressive narrowing and hardening of the arteries caused by age, high cholesterol, smoking, and/or other factors.
10. **c** An inflammation of the veins is called phlebitis.

Chapter 15 Practice Questions

1. **d** The function of lymph is to drain excess interstitial fluid, to transport lipids and vitamins, and to protect the body through the immune response.
2. **c** Lymphocytes are also known as B and T cells.
3. **d** Immunity acquired as the result of a vaccine is called active artificially acquired immunity.
4. **a** Small protein hormones that regulate many cell functions are called cytokines.
5. **c** The popliteal lymph nodes are located behind the knee.
6. **c** A malignant illness that begins with the infection of one lymph node is Hodgkin's disease.
7. **c** The lymphatic tissues that are covered by a membrane and located on either side of the throat are the tonsils.
8. **c** Fluid accumulation resulting in swelling is known as edema.
9. **a** An enlargement of the spleen is called splenomegaly.
10. **b** AIDS is the acronym for acquired immunodeficiency syndrome.

Chapter 16 Practice Questions

1. **b** The study of the lungs is called pulmonology.
2. **d** The "voice box" is the larynx.
3. **b** The air left in the lungs after a maximum exhalation is called residual volume.
4. **c** Small sacs in the lungs that fill with air are the alveoli.
5. **b** The dome-shaped muscle between the thoracic and abdominal cavities that controls breathing by relaxing and contracting is the diaphragm.
6. **d** ARDS is the acronym for acute respiratory distress syndrome.

7. **c** Metabolic reactions produce an excess of carbon dioxide, which must be eliminated quickly from the body.

8. **c** The larger air passages in the lungs are the bronchi.

9. **c** The exchange of gases between the air spaces in the lungs and the blood in the pulmonary capillaries is referred to as external respiration.

10. **d** The trachea is commonly known as the windpipe.

Chapter 17 Practice Questions

1. **a** The study of the digestive system is known as gastroenterology.

2. **d** Bile is secreted by the liver.

3. **b** The adult large intestine is approximately 5 feet in length.

4. **c** Mastication is the process of chewing food.

5. **b** The opening from the stomach to the intestine is the pylorus.

6. **d** Aphthous ulcers occur in the mouth.

7. **c** Gingivae are the gums of the mouth.

8. **b** Part of the stomach protruding through the diaphragm is a hiatal hernia.

9. **d** Binging and purging is known as bulimia nervosa.

10. **b** Borborygmus is caused by gas moving through the intestines.

Chapter 18 Practice Questions

1. **c** The sac that holds urine before it is expelled from the body is the bladder.

2. **b** There are two ureters in the body.

3. **b** In males, the tube that carries semen on its way out of the body is the urethra.

4. **c** Renal calculi are kidney stones.

5. **b** The tubes that transport urine from the kidneys to the bladder are the ureters.

6. **b** Ketones are metabolic byproducts of fat metabolism.

7. **d** Dialysis is a mechanical filtering of the blood caused by kidney failure.

8. **c** The condition of too many nitrogenous waste products left in the blood is known as azotemia.

9. **c** Frequent night-time urination is referred to as nocturia.

10. **a** The structures of the urinary system are the kidneys, ureters, bladder, and urethra.

Chapter 19 Practice Questions

1. **c** Gonads refer to both ovaries and testes.

2. **d** An autosome is a chromosome that has nothing to do with sex typing.

3. **b** Examples of secondary sex characteristics include the development of breasts.

4. **d** The most common bacterial sexually transmitted disease is chlamydia.

5. **d** Genital herpes is caused by a virus.

6. **a** The abnormal growth of the fetus somewhere other than in the uterus is called an ectopic pregnancy.

7. **b** The pair of structures near the prostate gland that manufacture semen are the seminal vesicles.

8. **c** Gametes are produced by both the ovaries and the testes.

9. **a** A diploid is a cell containing all the genetic material.

10. **d** Menarche is the onset of menstruation.

Chapter 20 Practice Questions

1. **c** Another term for the inner ear is the labyrinth.

2. **d** The main muscle responsible for any movement is the agonist.

3. **a** Proprioception allows us to move without thinking about it.

4. **c** Ergonomics is concerned with human factors pertaining to the environment.

5. **a** The three laws of motion were identified by Sir Isaac Newton.

6. **d** The factors that affect how/how much a bone is going to move are the position of the joint, the effort required, and the resistance encountered.

7. **d** The rarest lever in the body is the first-class lever.

8. **d** Improper biomechanics can cause injury, poor posture, carpal tunnel syndrome, and many other problems.

9. **c** Kinesthesia is the sensory perception of muscle movement.

10. **d** The ball of the foot is a second-class lever.

Chapter 21 Practice Questions

1. **c** Yin and yang are the opposite principles of the universe.

2. **b** Prana is a Sanskrit word that means "life force."

3. **c** The hara is located just below the navel.

4. **a** The path that is followed by Sushumna goes up the center of the spine.

5. **d** For clients who need to do gentle stretching exercises at home, you might suggest Tai Chi.

6. **b** Kapha dosha is described as wet, cold, and heavy, and corresponds to the element of water.

7. **a** Nadis and strotas are both channels.

8. **c** Wu-Hsing is the Chinese term for The Five Elements.

9. **b** To state that a point on the body is jitsu means that it is an area lacking in energy.

10. **d** In Ayurvedic massage, energy points are referred to as marmas.

Chapter 22 Practice Questions

1. **a** The term meridian is used to describe an energy pathway.

2. **c** There are 12 primary meridians.

3. **a** The conception vessel and governing vessel are referred to as extraordinary meridians.

4. **c** The liver is considered a yin organ.

5. **c** Chi circulates through the organs every 12 hours.

6. **d** The two meridians that do not have any element associated with them are the central meridian and the governing meridian.

7. **b** The central meridian is also referred to as the conception vessel.

8. **c** The lung meridian is actually paired with the large intestine meridian.

9. **d** The heart governor meridian is paired with the small intestine meridian.

10. **b** The meridian point that is referred to as the great eliminator is LI 4.

Chapter 23 Practice Questions

1. **d** The chakras are associated with endocrine glands.

2. **c** The chakra that is associated with perception is the third eye chakra.

3. **d** There are seven primary chakras.

4. **a** The chakra that is associated with the color green is the heart chakra.

5. **c** The throat chakra is associated with communication.

6. **a** Releasing waste from the body is associated with the base chakra.

7. **d** Chakras are associated with emotions, certain glands, and colors.

8. **a** The root chakra is associated with the sense of smell.

9. **d** Indigo is associated with the third eye chakra.

10. **a** The thyroid gland is associated with the throat chakra.

Chapter 24 Practice Questions

1. **a** S: Whatever the client states is recorded under "subjective."

2. **d** All of the above can be used to make a postural assessment, including a plumb line, a grid, or two pieces of tape on the wall.

3. **d** SOAP is the acronym for subjective, objective, assessment, plan.

4. **a** Informed consent should be obtained before doing any work on any client.

5. **d** Suggest that he see a doctor for a diagnosis anytime you observe a potentially harmful condition, making it plain that you are not offering a diagnosis.

6. **b** Touching and feeling the muscles for signs of tautness or trauma is referred to as palpation.

7. **a** Call the doctor before doing massage anytime you are confronted with a condition that you are not familiar with, particularly if the client does not have information to offer.

8. **b** Shoes that are badly worn on the outside of the heel are an indication of an eversion.

9. **c** When a client experiences an emotional release on the table, you should be present with them and act the part of a concerned listener.

10. **b** Subjective information is obtained by listening to the client.

Chapter 25 Practice Questions

1. **a** Interview the client a little more thoroughly to find out what, if any, complications he has and proceed with the massage in the normal manner, observing all universal precautions.

2. **b** If you have a bad cold, you should call your clients and reschedule them. "First, do no harm" includes not making people sick.

3. **a** Disinfecting everything with a germicide before the next client arrives is the safe way to proceed.

4. **c** Universal precautions should be observed with every client.

5. **d** A client who has a rash of unknown origin should not be massaged without a doctor's permission.

6. **c** If you sneeze while you are giving someone a massage, you should excuse yourself to go wash your hands, unless you were able to contort yourself so that both hands remained on the client's body while you turned away for the sneeze.

7. **d** You should wash your hands before and after eating, before and after each client, after handling laundry at the office, after using the restroom, and any other time as necessary.

8. **b** It is wise for massage therapists to be trained in CPR and first aid because they might have to be a first responder.

9. **d** The purpose of proper draping is to respect the modesty of the client, to protect the integrity of the therapist, and to keep the client warm.

10. **b** Explain to clients that draping is a law, as well as a safety precaution, and you are obligated to abide by the law.

Chapter 26 Practice Questions

1. **c** Reschedule any client who has a fever.

2. **c** Put her on the table and use gentle holding techniques and/or energy work. She has already decided to ignore the doctor, so your calling him will not make a difference, and gentle holding and/or energy work will not cause any harm.

3. **d** The popliteal triangle is located behind the knee.

4. **d** Thrombosis is another term for blood clot.

5. **b** A client who has had recent radiation therapy may be contraindicated for massage because of the effect of radiation on the skeletal system.

6. **c** Endangerment sites are places on the body that should be avoided because the veins, arteries, and/or nerves are superficial.

7. **c** Call her doctor (with her permission) to be able to make a more informed decision. Your primary concern is your and her safety.

8. **d** You should never massage a client who is under the influence of drugs or alcohol because the client may not be in control of himself, may say or do something inappropriate, or may accuse you of saying or doing something inappropriate.

9. **b** The axillary area (the armpit) is an endangerment site.

10. **c** Conduct a thorough interview, filling out the form as you go along, and check her blood pressure; if it is normal, go ahead with the massage.

Chapter 27 Practice Questions

1. **d** To assess a client's range of motion, you could put him through a series of joint mobilizations.

2. **a** To get the client acclimated to your touch and to warm up the muscle, you should begin bodywork sessions with effleurage.

3. **b** A client who has an area of inflammation due to a torn muscle would benefit from cryotherapy.

4. **d** Ballistic stretching is not a good technique for any use.

5. **a** The active assisted technique in which the muscle is stretched into resistance and then held for 10 seconds, followed by the client holding an isometric contraction for 5 seconds, is called the PNF technique, for proprioceptive neuromuscular facilitation.

6. **a** The technique that involves pumping is called compression.

7. **d** The technique that could be used to loosen congestion in the respiratory tract is called tapotement.

8. **b** Applying traction to the leg of a client who is lying supine is an example of passive stretching because the client is not doing anything to help.

9. **a** The therapist applying an unassisted stretch to the client would be equivalent to a passive static stretch.

10. **a** Hydrotherapy has the potential to affect the body in four ways, chemically, mechanically, thermally, and hydrostatically.

Chapter 28 Practice Questions

1. **c** Trager, Feldenkrais, and Alexander Technique all contain a component of movement on the part of the client.

2. **d** Swedish massage is the best modality for a client who wants a relaxation massage.

3. **d** Reiki is a modality in which the practitioner channels universal life energy to the client.

4. **d** Upledger and Sutherland are both known for their work in craniosacral therapy.

5. **b** Thai massage includes therapist-assisted yoga positionings.

6. **d** Therapeutic Touch would benefit a client who desires energy work instead of massage.

7. **c** Orthopedic massage is a rehabilitative technique for helping a client who is recovering from a bone injury.

8. **c** Auntie Margaret is associated with Lomi-Lomi.

9. **c** Visceral manipulation is aimed at releasing adhesions around the internal organs.

10. **c** Per Henrik Ling is credited with bringing Swedish massage to the United States.

Chapter 29 Practice Questions

1. **d** Tell them both politely that your code of ethics prohibits you from such behavior and in the interest of keeping your therapeutic relationship, you are not going to talk about the other. If they refuse to accept that, you will have to terminate them as clients.

2. **a** Tell him in no uncertain terms that you do therapeutic massage and do not have personal relationships with clients or share personal information. Put an immediate stop to problems of this nature. Ambiguity on your part could be perceived as assent.

3. **a** Step back behind the door where you can't see her and loudly say you'll be in when she gets under the sheet.

4. **c** Suggest that she seek counseling for the stress. Let a mental health professional be the one to tell her she enjoys playing the martyr.

5. **b** Call him immediately after the session to discuss the matter, without divulging the client's name. Avoid judgment and recrimination, and stress that as a colleague these accusations are a cause for concern.

6. **a** Listen and be compassionate when a client discusses personal matters with you. Don't offer unsolicited advice.

7. **c** You have just violated the client's boundaries. You may ask if you can unhook it, but you should not just assume it is okay to do it.

8. **b** Tell her politely that you cannot talk about your clients—and that you wouldn't talk about her.

9. **a** Send a formal complaint to the massage board. If you are in a state that has licensure laws, you are obligated to do just that.

10. **a** You have violated the rule of confidentiality.

Chapter 30 Practice Questions

1. **b** If you are working as an independent contractor, the IRS requires that you file quarterly self-employment taxes.

2. **c** If you are a business owner who employs other therapists, pays them by the hour, and provides them with benefits, you will be giving them a W-2 form at the end of the tax year.

3. **a** The best course of action is to get another therapist to cover her appointments if at all possible. A bawling therapist will not make a good impression on clients.

4. **c** A mission statement is a written expression of the goals and purposes of a business.

5. **d** To protect yourself from a lawsuit, you should have liability insurance.

6. **b** The main purpose of a code of ethics is to provide parameters for a safe and comfortable therapeutic relationship.

7. **a** If a massage practitioner with a license in one state moves to another state and a license is granted based on the license from the previous state, it is called reciprocity.

8. **c** A practitioner who receives referrals from a physician should always provide the doctor with progress notes (and a thank you note would be nice, too).

9. **a** If you are the sole owner of a business, it is referred to as a proprietorship.

10. **a** The cost of continuing education after you have your license would be the only legitimate tax-deductible business expense. Training for a new career is not deductible, nor are any costs associated with it under normal circumstances. Training that is meant to enhance your present career (for instance, if you are already a physical therapist) is generally deductible. Check with your tax professional.

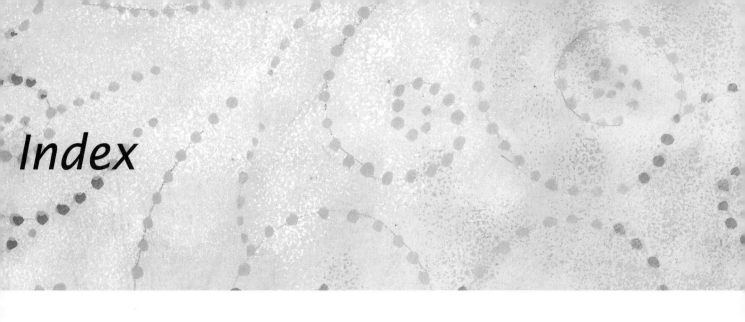

Index

Page numbers in *italics* denote figure; those followed by t denote table.